LARGE SIMPLE TRIALS AND KNOWLEDGE GENERATION IN A LEARNING HEALTH SYSTEM

Workshop Summary

Claudia Grossmann, Julia Sanders, and Rebecca A. English, *Rapporteurs*

Roundtable on Value & Science-Driven Health Care

Forum on Drug Discovery, Development, and Translation

Board on Health Sciences Policy

INSTITUTE OF MEDICINE
OF THE NATIONAL ACADEMIES

THE NATIONAL ACADEMIES PRESS
Washington, D.C.
www.nap.edu

THE NATIONAL ACADEMIES PRESS 500 Fifth Street, NW Washington, DC 20001

NOTICE: The workshop that is the subject of this workshop summary was approved by the Governing Board of the National Research Council, whose members are drawn from the councils of the National Academy of Sciences, the National Academy of Engineering, and the Institute of Medicine.

This activity was supported by contracts between the National Academy of Sciences and the U.S. Department of Health and Human Services (Contract No. N01-OD-4-2139 TO #203 and HHSN26300023 [Under Base No. HHSN263201200074I] and Contract No. N01-OD-4-2139 TO #276; HHSF22301026T [Under Base No. HHSF223200810020I]), AbbVie Inc., Agency for Healthcare Research and Quality, American Diabetes Association, American Society for Microbiology, Amgen Inc., Association of American Medical Colleges, AstraZeneca, Blue Shield of California, Blue Shield of California Foundation, Bristol-Myers Squibb, Burroughs Wellcome Fund, Celtic Therapeutics, LLLP, Centers for Medicare & Medicaid Services, Critical Path Institute, Doris Duke Charitable Foundation, Eli Lilly and Company, Epic Systems, Inc., FasterCures, Friends of Cancer Research, GlaxoSmithKline, Gordon and Betty Moore Foundation, Health Resources and Services Administration, Hospital Corporation of America, Inc., Johnson & Johnson, Kaiser Permanente (East Bay Community Foundation), March of Dimes Foundation, Merck & Co., Inc., Novartis Pharmaceuticals Corporation, Partners HealthCare, Patient-Centered Outcomes Research Institute, Pfizer Inc., Premier, Sanofi, United Health Foundation, and WellPoint, Inc. The views presented in this publication do not necessarily reflect the views of the organizations or agencies that provided support for the activity.

International Standard Book Number-13: 978-0-309-28911-5
International Standard Book Number-10: 0-309-28911-4

Additional copies of this workshop summary are available for sale from the National Academies Press, 500 Fifth Street, NW, Keck 360, Washington, DC 20001; (800) 624-6242 or (202) 334-3313; http://www.nap.edu.

For more information about the Institute of Medicine, visit the IOM home page at: www.iom.edu.

The serpent has been a symbol of long life, healing, and knowledge among almost all cultures and religions since the beginning of recorded history. The serpent adopted as a logotype by the Institute of Medicine is a relief carving from ancient Greece, now held by the Staatliche Museen in Berlin.

Suggested citation: IOM (Institute of Medicine). 2013. *Large simple trials and knowledge generation in a learning health system: Workshop summary.* Washington, DC: The National Academies Press.

"Knowing is not enough; we must apply.
Willing is not enough; we must do."

—Goethe

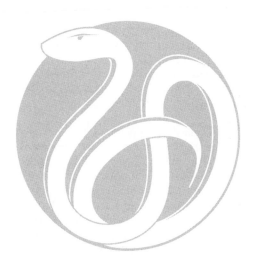

INSTITUTE OF MEDICINE
OF THE NATIONAL ACADEMIES

Advising the Nation. Improving Health.

THE NATIONAL ACADEMIES
Advisers to the Nation on Science, Engineering, and Medicine

The **National Academy of Sciences** is a private, nonprofit, self-perpetuating society of distinguished scholars engaged in scientific and engineering research, dedicated to the furtherance of science and technology and to their use for the general welfare. Upon the authority of the charter granted to it by the Congress in 1863, the Academy has a mandate that requires it to advise the federal government on scientific and technical matters. Dr. Ralph J. Cicerone is president of the National Academy of Sciences.

The **National Academy of Engineering** was established in 1964, under the charter of the National Academy of Sciences, as a parallel organization of outstanding engineers. It is autonomous in its administration and in the selection of its members, sharing with the National Academy of Sciences the responsibility for advising the federal government. The National Academy of Engineering also sponsors engineering programs aimed at meeting national needs, encourages education and research, and recognizes the superior achievements of engineers. Dr. C. D. Mote, Jr., is president of the National Academy of Engineering.

The **Institute of Medicine** was established in 1970 by the National Academy of Sciences to secure the services of eminent members of appropriate professions in the examination of policy matters pertaining to the health of the public. The Institute acts under the responsibility given to the National Academy of Sciences by its congressional charter to be an adviser to the federal government and, upon its own initiative, to identify issues of medical care, research, and education. Dr. Harvey V. Fineberg is president of the Institute of Medicine.

The **National Research Council** was organized by the National Academy of Sciences in 1916 to associate the broad community of science and technology with the Academy's purposes of furthering knowledge and advising the federal government. Functioning in accordance with general policies determined by the Academy, the Council has become the principal operating agency of both the National Academy of Sciences and the National Academy of Engineering in providing services to the government, the public, and the scientific and engineering communities. The Council is administered jointly by both Academies and the Institute of Medicine. Dr. Ralph J. Cicerone and Dr. C. D. Mote, Jr., are chair and vice chair, respectively, of the National Research Council.

www.national-academies.org

PLANNING COMMITTEE FOR THE WORKSHOP ON LARGE SIMPLE TRIALS AND KNOWLEDGE GENERATION IN A LEARNING SYSTEM[1]

DAVID L. DEMETS (*Co-Chair*), Professor, Biostatistics and Medical Informatics, University of Wisconsin School of Public Health

RICHARD E. KUNTZ (*Co-Chair*), Senior Vice President and Chief Scientific, Clinical, and Regulatory Officer, Medtronic

WILLIAM H. CROWN, President, HEOR and Late Phase Research, OPTUMInsight Life Sciences

JEFFREY M. DRAZEN, Editor-in-Chief, *New England Journal of Medicine*

RALPH I. HORWITZ, Senior Vice President, Clinical Sciences Evaluation, GlaxoSmithKline

PETRA KAUFMANN, Director, Office of Clinical Research, National Institute of Neurological Disorders and Stroke

JUDITH M. KRAMER, Senior Scientific Advisor, Clinical Trials Transformation Initiative, Duke Translational Medicine Institute

MICHAEL S. LAUER, Director, Division of Cardiovascular Sciences, National Heart, Lung, and Blood Institute

JOANN E. MANSON, Professor of Medicine, Harvard Medical School

JOHN J. ORLOFF, Chief Medical Officer and Senior Vice President, Global Development, U.S. Medical and Drug Regulatory Affairs, Novartis Pharmaceuticals Corporation

ERIC D. PETERSON, Professor of Medicine, Division of Cardiology, Duke University Medical School

RICHARD PLATT, Chair, Population Medicine, Harvard Medical School

JOE V. SELBY, Executive Director, Patient-Centered Outcomes Research Institute

RACHEL E. SHERMAN, Director, Office of Medical Policy, Center for Drug Evaluation and Research, U.S. Food and Drug Administration

JOSE M. VEGA, Vice President, Global Safety, Amgen Inc.

---

[1] Institute of Medicine planning committees are solely responsible for organizing the workshop, identifying topics, and choosing speakers. The responsibility for the published workshop summary rests with the workshop rapporteurs and the institution.

ROUNDTABLE ON VALUE & SCIENCE-DRIVEN HEALTH CARE[1]

MARK B. McCLELLAN (*Chair*), Senior Fellow and Director, Health Care Innovation and Value Initiative, The Brookings Institution

RAYMOND BAXTER, Senior Vice President, Community, Benefit, Research and Health Policy, Kaiser Permanente

DAVID BLUMENTHAL, President, The Commonwealth Fund

BRUCE G. BODAKEN, Former Chairman and Chief Executive Officer, Blue Shield of California

PAUL CHEW, Chief Science Officer and Chief Medical Officer, Sanofi U.S.

FRANCIS COLLINS, Director, National Institutes of Health (Ex Officio) (*designee:* **Kathy Hudson**)

HELEN DARLING, President, National Business Group on Health

SUSAN DEVORE, Chief Executive Officer, Premier, Inc.

JUDITH FAULKNER, Founder and Chief Executive Officer, Epic Health Systems

THOMAS R. FRIEDEN, Director, Centers for Disease Control and Prevention (Ex Officio) (*designee:* **James Galloway**)

PATRICIA A. GABOW, Former Chief Executive Officer, Denver Health

ATUL GAWANDE, General and Endocrine Surgeon, Brigham and Women's Hospital

GARY L. GOTTLIEB, President and Chief Executive Officer, Partners HealthCare

JAMES A. GUEST, President and Chief Executive Officer, Consumers Union

GEORGE C. HALVORSON, Chairman and Chief Executive Officer, Kaiser Permanente

MARGARET A. HAMBURG, Commissioner, U.S. Food and Drug Administration (Ex Officio) (*designee:* **Peter Lurie**)

JAMES HEYWOOD, Cofounder and Chairman, PatientsLikeMe

RALPH I. HORWITZ, Senior Vice President, Clinical Evaluation Sciences, GlaxoSmithKline

PAUL HUDSON, Executive Vice President, AstraZeneca

BRENT C. JAMES, Chief Quality Officer, Intermountain Healthcare

CRAIG JONES, Director, Vermont Blueprint for Health

GARY KAPLAN, Chairman and Chief Executive Officer, Virginia Mason Health System

---

[1] Institute of Medicine forums and roundtables do not issue, review, or approve individual documents. The responsibility for the published workshop summary rests with the workshop rapporteurs and the institution.

IOM Staff

KATHERINE BURNS, Program Assistant
CLAUDIA GROSSMANN, Senior Program Officer
DIEDTRA HENDERSON, Program Officer
ELIZABETH JOHNSTON, Program Assistant
ELIZABETH ROBINSON, Research Associate
VALERIE ROHRBACH, Senior Program Assistant
JULIA SANDERS, Senior Program Assistant (through August 2013)
ROBERT SAUNDERS, Senior Program Officer
BARRET ZIMMERMANN, Program Assistant (through October 2013)
J. MICHAEL McGINNIS, Senior Scholar, Executive Director, Roundtable
    on Value & Science-Driven Health Care

FORUM ON DRUG DISCOVERY, DEVELOPMENT, AND TRANSLATION[1]

JEFFREY M. DRAZEN (*Co-Chair*), Editor-in-Chief, *New England Journal of Medicine*

STEVEN K. GALSON (*Co-Chair*), Global Regulatory Vice President, Amgen Inc.

RUSS BIAGIO ALTMAN, The Kenneth Fong Professor of Bioengineering, Genetics, Medicine, and (by courtesy) Computer Science, Stanford University

MARGARET ANDERSON, Executive Director, FasterCures

HUGH AUCHINCLOSS, Deputy Director, National Institute of Allergy and Infectious Diseases

CHRISTOPHER P. AUSTIN, Director, National Center for Advancing Translational Sciences

ANN C. BONHAM, Chief Scientific Officer, Association of American Medical Colleges

LINDA BRADY, Director, Division of Neuroscience and Basic Behavioral Science, National Institute of Mental Health

GAIL H. CASSELL, Visiting Professor, Department of Social Medicine and Global Medicine, Harvard Medical School

PETER B. CORR, Cofounder, Managing General Partner, Auven Therapeutics, LLP

ANDREW M. DAHLEM, Vice President and Chief Operating Officer, Lilly Research Laboratories, Eli Lilly and Company

JAMES H. DOROSHOW, Deputy Director for Clinical and Translational Research, Division of Cancer Treatment and Diagnosis, National Cancer Institute

GARY L. FILERMAN, President, Atlas Health Foundation

MARK J. GOLDBERGER, Divisional Vice President, Regulatory Policy and Intelligence, Pharmaceutical Products Group, Abbott Pharmaceuticals

HARRY B. GREENBERG, Senior Associate Dean for Research and Joseph D. Grant Professor of Medicine, Microbiology, and Immunology, Stanford University School of Medicine

PETER K. HONIG, Global Vice President, Regulatory Affairs, AstraZeneca

KATHY L. HUDSON, Deputy Director for Science, Outreach, and Policy, National Institutes of Health

---

[1] Institute of Medicine forums and roundtables do not issue, review, or approve individual documents. The responsibility for the published workshop summary rests with the workshop rapporteurs and the institution.

LYNN D. HUDSON, Chief Science Officer, Critical Path Institute

S. CLAIBORNE JOHNSTON, Professor of Neurology and Epidemiology, Associate Vice Chancellor of Research, and Director, Clinical and Translational Science Institute, University of California, San Francisco

MICHAEL KATZ, Senior Advisor, Transdisciplinary Research, March of Dimes Foundation

PETRA KAUFMANN, Director, Office of Clinical Research, National Institute of Neurological Disorders and Stroke

JACK D. KEENE, James B. Duke Professor of Molecular Genetics and Microbiology, Duke University Medical Center

RUSTY KELLEY, Program Officer, Burroughs Wellcome Fund

RONALD L. KRALL, Associate Fellow, University of Pennsylvania Center for Bioethics

FREDA C. LEWIS-HALL, Executive Vice President and Chief Medical Officer, Pfizer Inc.

CAROL MIMURA, Assistant Vice Chancellor for Intellectual Property & Industry Research Alliances, University of California, Berkeley

BERNARD H. MUNOS, Founder, InnoThink Center for Research in Biomedical Innovation

ELIZABETH (BETSY) MYERS, Program Director for Medical Research, Doris Duke Charitable Foundation

JOHN J. ORLOFF, Chief Medical Officer and Senior Vice President, Global Development, U.S. Medical and Drug Regulatory Affairs, Novartis Pharmaceuticals Corporation

ROBERT E. RATNER, Chief Scientific Medical Officer, American Diabetes Association

MICHAEL ROSENBLATT, Executive Vice President and Chief Medical Officer, Merck & Co., Inc.

JAMES S. SHANNON, Chief Medical Officer, GlaxoSmithKline

JANET SHOEMAKER, Director, Office of Public Affairs, American Society for Microbiology

ELLEN V. SIGAL, Chair and Founder, Friends of Cancer Research

LANA R. SKIRBOLL, Vice President, Academic and Scientific Affairs, Sanofi

BRIAN L. STROM, Executive Vice Dean for Institutional Affairs and Professor, University of Pennsylvania Perelman School of Medicine

JANET TOBIAS, President, Sierra/Tango Productions, Ikana Media

JOANNE WALDSTREICHER, Chief Medical Officer, Johnson & Johnson

JANET WOODCOCK, Director, Center for Drug Evaluation and Research, U.S. Food and Drug Administration

IOM Staff

ANNE B. CLAIBORNE, Forum Director
REBECCA A. ENGLISH, Associate Program Officer
ELIZABETH F. C. TYSON, Research Associate
ROBIN GUYSE, Senior Program Assistant
ANDREW M. POPE, Director, Board on Health Sciences Policy

Reviewers

This workshop summary has been reviewed in draft form by individuals chosen for their diverse perspectives and technical expertise, in accordance with procedures approved by the National Research Council's Report Review Committee. The purpose of this independent review is to provide candid and critical comments that will assist the institution in making its published workshop summary as sound as possible and to ensure that the workshop summary meets institutional standards for objectivity, evidence, and responsiveness to the study charge. The review comments and draft manuscript remain confidential to protect the integrity of the process. We wish to thank the following individuals for their review of this workshop summary:

Stefan James, Uppsala University Hospital
Elliott Levy, Bristol-Myers Squibb
Sean Tunis, Center for Medical Technology Policy
Paul J. Wallace, Optum Labs

Although the reviewers listed above have provided many constructive comments and suggestions, they did not see the final draft of the workshop summary before its release. The review of this workshop summary was overseen by **Joel Kupersmith,** Veterans Health Administration. Appointed by the Institute of Medicine, he was responsible for making certain that an independent examination of this workshop summary was carried out in accordance with institutional procedures and that all review comments were carefully considered. Responsibility for the final content of this workshop summary rests entirely with the rapporteurs and the institution.

Preface

The current paradigms for effectiveness research and drug development face increasingly acute challenges in cost, timing, and applicability, given their reliance on classic randomized controlled trials. Opportunities to engage these challenges by the use of large simple trial (LST) designs and the integration of research at the point of care prompted the Institute of Medicine's Roundtable on Value & Science-Driven Health Care (the Roundtable) and the Forum on Drug Discovery, Development, and Translation (the Forum) to convene a workshop, Large Simple Trials and Knowledge Generation in a Learning Health System, which is summarized in this publication.

Experts from a wide range of disciplines—including health information technology, research funding, clinical research methods, statistics, patients, product development, medical product regulation, and clinical outcomes research—met to marshal a better understanding of the issues, options, and approaches to accelerating the use of LSTs. This publication summarizes discussions on the potential of LSTs to improve the speed and practicality of knowledge generation for medical decision making and medical product development, including efficacy and effectiveness assessments, in a continuously learning health system.

The work of the Roundtable is focused on moving toward a continuously learning health system, one in which every care encounter is an opportunity for learning and evidence is applied to ensure and improve best care practices. Since its inception in 2006, the Roundtable has set out to help realize this vision through the support, involvement, and activities of senior leadership from key stakeholders in the health care system.

Since its creation in 2005, the Forum has provided a platform for dialogue and collaboration among thought leaders and stakeholders in government, academia, industry, foundations, and patient advocacy. Since 2009, the Forum has convened an ongoing initiative dedicated to addressing the challenges facing the U.S. clinical trials enterprise by bringing together the broad range of clinical research stakeholders to surface potentially transformative strategies to improve the efficiency and effectiveness of clinical trials. The Forum's public meetings focus substantial public attention on critical areas of drug discovery, development, and translation and in doing so serve to educate the policy community about issues where science and policy intersect.

Building on this groundwork, the objectives of this workshop were to explore acceleration of the use of LSTs to improve the speed and practicality of knowledge generation for medical decision making and medical product development; consider the concepts of LST design, examples of successful LSTs, the relative advantages of LSTs, and the infrastructure needed to build LST capacity as a routine function of care; identify structural, cultural, and regulatory barriers hindering the development of an enhanced LST capacity; discuss needs and strategies in building public demand for and participation in LSTs; and consider near-term strategies for accelerating progress in the uptake of LSTs in the United States.

Multiple individuals donated valuable time toward the development of this publication. We acknowledge and offer strong appreciation to the contributors to this publication for their presence at the workshop and their efforts to further develop their presentations into the summaries contained in this publication. We are especially indebted to those who provided counsel by serving on the planning committee for this workshop.

A number of Roundtable and Forum staff played instrumental roles in coordinating the workshop and translating the workshop proceedings into this summary, including Claudia Grossmann, Anne Claiborne, Julia Sanders, Rebecca A. English, Elizabeth Johnston, Elizabeth Tyson, Valerie Rohrbach, Robin Guyse, Barret Zimmermann, Rob Saunders, Diedtra Henderson, and Elizabeth Robinson. Finally, we thank Daniel Bethea, Marton Cavani, Laura Harbold DeStefano, and Chelsea Frakes for helping to coordinate various aspects of review, production, and publication.

A fundamental component of a learning health system is the ability to improve the speed and practicality of knowledge generation. The increased use of LSTs that rely on larger, more representative populations, and optimize data collection could serve to speed the necessary transformation. We believe that *Large Simple Trials and Knowledge Generation in a Learning Health System: Workshop Summary* will be a valuable resource in informing this transformation.

David L. DeMets
Planning Committee Co-Chair
Professor
University of Wisconsin School of Public Health

Richard E. Kuntz
Planning Committee Co-Chair
Senior Vice President and
Chief Scientific, Clinical, and Regulatory Officer
Medtronic

J. Michael McGinnis
Senior Scholar
Executive Director
Roundtable on Value & Science-Driven Health Care
Institute of Medicine

Andrew M. Pope
Director
Board on Health Sciences Policy
Institute of Medicine

Contents

1

Introduction[1]

Randomized clinical trials (RCTs) are often referred to as the "gold standard" of clinical research. However, it is well documented that, in its current state, the U.S. clinical trials enterprise faces substantial challenges to the efficient and effective conduct of research (IOM, 2012a; Sung et al., 2003). Streamlined approaches to RCTs, such as large simple trials (LSTs), may provide opportunities for progress on these challenges.

Clinical trials support the development of new medical products and the evaluation of existing products by generating knowledge about safety and efficacy in pre- and post-marketing settings and serve to inform medical decision making and medical product development. Although well-designed and well-implemented clinical trials can provide robust evidence, a gap exists between the evidence needs of a continuously learning health system, in which all medical decisions are based on the best available evidence, and the reality, in which the generation of timely and practical evidence faces significant barriers.

Escalating costs, lengthy timelines, and the inability to regularly apply the evidence from clinical trials to broader populations are some of the challenges facing the U.S. clinical trials enterprise. Clinical trials are frequently conducted in a one-off manner: resources, staff, and research

---

[1] The planning committee's role was limited to planning the workshop, and the workshop summary has been prepared by the workshop rapporteurs as a factual summary of what occurred at the workshop. Statements, recommendations, and opinions expressed are those of individual presenters and participants and are not necessarily endorsed or verified by the Roundtable, the Forum, or the Institute of Medicine, and they should not be construed as reflecting any group consensus.

participants are brought together for a single study and subsequently disbanded, increasing time and costs across the research enterprise. The complexity of individual clinical trials is also a barrier to the efficient generation of evidence. Clinical trial protocols (i.e., the blueprint for how a study will be conducted) involve increasing amounts of tests, procedures, and data collection to support noncore endpoints (Tufts Center for the Study of Drug Development, 2012). The inclusion of these additional components heightens the workload for clinical study staff, increases overall study time and costs, and increases the burden on participants.

Although challenges to the traditional RCT exist, a diverse portfolio of research methods, including innovative approaches to RCTs, is warranted to address evidence needs across the learning health care system—for example, to inform medical providers treating patients with multiple conditions, researchers comparing the effectiveness of medical treatments, newly diagnosed patients exploring treatment options, and medical product developers pursuing new treatments for unmet medical needs. Innovative approaches include the use of streamlined designs, such as those used for LSTs; trials performed in settings that more closely mirror real-world settings, such as pragmatic trials; trials embedded in health care delivery settings, such as point-of-care trials; and trials that are modified while they are in progress, such as adaptive trials, among others.

The simplified design and the use of large, diverse populations to study an intervention make LSTs useful for scientific inquiries of commonly used therapies for which the difference in treatment effects is unknown. This is in contrast to, for example, an early stage (Phase I) clinical trial to test the tolerability of a new medicine. Such a trial requires a small group of patients with a particular disease profile and would be less well-suited to an LST type of design. According to Peto et al. (1995), LSTs are designed to detect small or moderate treatment effects through the use of a simplified clinical trial design that deploys randomization to minimize bias and random error.

During the workshop, the term "LST" was used broadly and encompassed trials with a number of different attributes. The attributes of LSTs discussed during the workshop include the following: LSTs have simple randomization; broad eligibility criteria leading to a large, diverse patient population and increased generalizability of the study results; enough trial participants to provide evidence on interventions with small to moderate effects; a focus on meaningful outcomes important to patient care; and a streamlined design that provides a mechanism for effectively and efficiently capturing outcomes.

Several examples of successful LSTs are available, including the Gruppo Italiano per lo Studio della Sopravvivenza nell'Infarto Miocardico (GISSI) trials, which evaluated patient survival after acute myocardial infarction. The GISSI trials employed protocols embedded in clinical practice, which allowed the participation of more than 60,000 patients and almost four out of every five coronary care units that existed in Italy at the time (GISSI, 2013). The involvement of such a large percentage of the country's cardiology clinics is credited with accelerating the uptake and implementation of the trials' results.

Significant opportunities exist to accelerate the use of LSTs to efficiently generate practical evidence for medical decision making and product development. Data for LSTs can be obtained from electronic health records (EHRs), whose increased adoption continues to be driven by the implementation of the Health Information Technology for Economic and Clinical Health Act, which pays incentives to hospitals or eligible office-based professionals if they demonstrate use of their EHRs in a meaningful way. With more than 40 percent of hospitals and office-based physicians employing at least a basic EHR system in 2012, the ability to collect research data in the course of regular care is greater than ever (RWJF, 2013). This could allow trials with streamlined data collection requirements to be supported by data captured in preexisting EHRs. For example, the Study of Technology to Accelerate Research (STAR) in Massachusetts (which is discussed in more detail in Chapter 3) successfully based its ongoing trial on childhood obesity screening and management strategies on the electronic medical records already in use at each of its 14 participating sites (Clinicaltrials.gov, 2012). STAR offers a strong example of how the EHR can be used as the foundation for LST design and implementation.

With the potential for such applicability and widespread use, LSTs present the opportunity, together with and as a complement to quasiexperimental methods, registries, and safety efforts, to improve the speed and practicality of knowledge generation, characteristics fundamental to a learning health care system. With the development of new technologies capable of acquiring, managing, linking, and analyzing large quantities of data, the potential for innovation in methods, including the ability to draw research insights from routine clinical care experiences more effectively, is growing. Moreover, the increased use of innovative methodologies, such as LSTs, and their incorporation into routine clinical care can allow more patients than ever to engage in research to improve health care delivery and outcomes. Through streamlined protocols, the electronic availability of trial tools and outcomes data, and capabilities for remote participation, every patient has the potential to be a contributor to the continuous learning process and improve not only the outcomes of treatment for that individual but also the outcomes for other patients with similar conditions. LSTs offer the potential to drive the transformation necessary to realize this vision.

To address these opportunities, as well as challenges, the Institute of Medicine's (IOM's) Roundtable on Value & Science-Driven Health Care (the Roundtable) and the Forum on Drug Discovery, Development, and

Translation (the Forum) convened a public workshop on November 26 and 27, 2012, titled Large Simple Trials and Knowledge Generation in a Learning Health System. A frequent theme raised in the workshops conducted for both the Roundtable and the Forum is that the cost, timing, and applicability limitations of the current effectiveness research and drug development paradigms, namely, a reliance on classic RCTs, become more acute daily. This workshop thus expanded on other workshops and discussions of the Forum to address the challenges facing the U.S. clinical trials enterprise and engage stakeholders in an open discussion of potentially transformative strategies to improve the efficiency and effectiveness of clinical trials, as summarized in Box 1-1. The workshop similarly expanded on the Roundtable's previous discussions and workshops on improving approaches to clinical effectiveness research, as summarized in Box 1-2, which it continues to foster through the discussions and products of the Clinical Effectiveness Research Innovation Collaborative.

WORKSHOP SCOPE AND OBJECTIVES

The workshop participants included a broad range of experts in clinical research, medical product development, patient advocacy, biostatistics, health information technology, clinical data standards, ethics, legal/regulatory issues, and health care payment and financing. The workshop was structured to highlight the pros and cons of the design characteristics of LSTs, explore the utility of LSTs on the basis of case studies of past successes, and consider the challenges and opportunities for accelerating the use of LSTs in the context of a U.S. clinical trials enterprise that could benefit from increased implementation of simplified and streamlined clinical trial designs that produce generalizable results.

In addition to drawing on a diverse array of perspectives on LST uptake, the workshop also explored infrastructure needs, the role of EHRs in LSTs, policies surrounding the enhanced use of LSTs, and the need for enhanced stakeholder engagement with health systems, clinicians, patients, and payers to successfully implement LSTs.

The workshop statement of task can be found in Box 1-3, and the stated meeting objectives were as follows:

- Explore acceleration of the use of LSTs to improve the speed and practicality of knowledge generation for medical decision making and medical product development;
- Consider the concepts of LST design, examples of successful LSTs, the relative advantages of LSTs, and the infrastructure needed to build LST capacity as a routine function of care;

BOX 1-1
Key Themes from Workshops Conducted for the
Forum on Drug Discovery, Development, and Translation

- *Identification of inefficiencies in the U.S. clinical trials enterprise.* High costs, extended trial timelines, high rates of investigator turnover, and low patient recruitment are a few challenges facing the conduct of clinical trials in the United States (IOM, 2010a, 2012a).
- *Research in the context of globalization.* Competition from other countries, where research costs are lower or governments are supporting growth in their indigenous medical research industry, is growing (IOM, 2010a, 2012a).
- *Transformative strategies to improve the efficiency of clinical trials.* Harmonization of regulatory standards and institutional processes, establishment of a national clinical trials infrastructure, and consideration of models to more effectively manage the nation's research portfolio could advance the efficiency and effectiveness of the research enterprise and ultimately improve patient care (IOM, 2012a).
- *Convergence of clinical research and clinical practice.* Incorporation of clinical research into the continuous quality improvement activities already undertaken by the health care system can help generate valid, reliable, and relevant evidence for medical practice (IOM, 2012a,b).
- *Patients and community health care providers as partners in clinical research.* The formation of collaborations between researchers, community health care providers, and patients early in the research process can facilitate the success of a clinical trial, from patient recruitment to the dissemination of trial results and assurance of the uptake of those results in clinical practice (IOM, 2012b).
- *Workforce and career development.* Greater attention to research in medical school could improve practitioners' attitudes toward research and attract young physicians to research careers. Similarly, placement of a higher value on the conduct of clinical trials in tenure decisions could enhance career ladders in research (IOM, 2012a).
- *Cultural and financial incentives.* Incentives for research may be provided and the efficiency of research may be increased if academic institutions and research organizations were encouraged to move beyond provincial systems in favor of greater efficiency (e.g., abandoning a site-specific institutional review board [IRB] for a centralized IRB model) and disincentives for research were corrected through the provision of more coverage under evidence development (from private payers as well as Medicare) (IOM, 2012a).

- Identify structural, cultural, and regulatory barriers hindering the development of an enhanced LST capacity and discuss needs and strategies in building public demand for and participation in LSTs; and
- Suggest near-term strategies for accelerating progress in the uptake of LSTs in the United States.

BOX 1-2
Key Themes from Workshops Conducted for the
Roundtable on Value & Science-Driven Health Care

- *Limitations to applicability of research results.* Current clinical studies are often designed to focus on people with just one condition, limiting their applicability to the increasing number people with multiple conditions (IOM, 2010b).
- *Inefficiencies related to the timeliness, cost, and volume of clinical research.* Each incremental unit of research time and money could contribute to confidence in the results but also carries greater opportunity costs (IOM, 2010b).
- *New research designs, tools, and analytics.* Innovative research designs and statistical techniques may accelerate the timeliness and level of research insights, helping to better target, tailor, and refine approaches (IOM, 2010b, 2011).
- *Incentives for innovation in clinical effectiveness research.* The use of new and emerging tools to draw clinical research closer to practice will also require innovative economic, regulatory, and clinician-patient cultural incentives for their application (IOM, 2010b).
- *Effectiveness research as a routine part of practice.* Learning from every element of the care process is the theoretical goal of a learning health care system. This means anchoring the focus of clinical effectiveness research planning and priority setting on the point of service—the patient–provider interface—and enlisting the patient as an advocate in the process (IOM, 2010b, 2011).
- *Transformational research potential of information technology.* Broad application and linkage of electronic health records afford the possibility of real-time clinical effectiveness research (IOM, 2010b, 2011).
- *Patients as central partners in the learning culture.* Taking full advantage of clinical records, even with blinded information, requires a strong level of understanding and support for the work and its importance to improving the quality of health care. (IOM, 2010b).
- *Continuous learning in all aspects of care.* This foundational principle of a learning health care system depends on system and culture change in each element of the care process with the potential to promote interest, activity, and involvement in the process of knowledge and evidence development, from health professions education to care delivery and payment (IOM, 2010b).

ORGANIZATION OF THE SUMMARY

This publication summarizes the proceedings of Large Simple Trials and Knowledge Generation in a Learning Health System, a joint workshop coordinated by the Roundtable and the Forum in 2012. Each chapter of this summary corresponds to a workshop session and includes a summary of key speaker themes from each presentation. A selection of key speaker themes from across all sessions can be found in Box 1-4.

BOX 1-3
Statement of Task

An ad hoc planning committee will plan and conduct a public workshop to explore acceleration of the use of large simple trials (LSTs) to improve the speed and practicality of knowledge generation for medical decision making and medical product development, including efficacy and effectiveness assessments, in a continuously learning health system. The committee will steer development of the agenda for the workshop, including selection of speakers and discussants. Workshop content will explore the concepts of LST design; examples of successful LSTs; the relative advantages of LSTs (in terms of cost and the utility of the results); the infrastructure needed to build LST capacity as a routine function of care; the structural, cultural, and regulatory barriers hindering the development of such an LST capacity; building public demand for and participation in LSTs; and identifying near-term strategies for accelerating progress.

BOX 1-4
Select Speaker Themes

- LSTs and greater patient involvement in research will be key to moving the U.S. health care system to a future in which every clinical encounter is an opportunity for learning (Michael S. Lauer).
- LSTs pose a series of challenges and opportunities for the clinical research enterprise. These include solidification of their external validity, better understanding of the implications for the detection of treatment heterogeneity and patient safety, and exploration of opportunities for greater integration of patient-reported outcomes (Ralph I. Horwitz).
- LSTs provide an opportunity to conduct cost-efficient research with clinical and policy relevance, as well as take advantage of emerging research methods and data sources for the benefit of population health (Niteesh K. Choudhry, P. J. Devereaux, Joann E. Manson, Elsie M. Taveras).
- LSTs provide an opportunity to bridge the gap between research activities and clinical practice by appropriately balancing the risks and benefits of research when the safety and effectiveness of routine clinical practices are often unknown (Ruth R. Faden).
- Technical challenges to LSTs have been addressed in large part, and policy and culture changes remain the primary challenges to increased LST uptake (Robert M. Califf).

Chapters 2 to 8 summarize the expert presentations at the workshop and are organized by thematic focus. Chapter 2 focuses on the current state and momentum of the LST enterprise. Chapter 3 looks at several examples of LSTs, emphasizing trade-offs in trial design and their impact on the research process and outcomes. Chapter 4 takes a look at the current state of trial complexity, strategies for increasing trial efficacy, and the perspective of the U.S. Food and Drug Administration. Chapter 5 addresses the infrastructure needs and barriers to the performance of more LSTs and discusses both the current state and future potential of the use of EHRs as platforms for LSTs. Chapter 6 delves into the real and perceived ethical and policy barriers to the greater use of LSTs, highlighting examples of ways in which such barriers have been confronted and suggesting components of a policy framework that would facilitate LSTs. Chapter 7 explores partnerships with stakeholders relevant to the increased use of LSTs, focusing on the elements of the greatest importance to patients, payers, clinicians, and health care systems in advancing the uptake of LSTs. Chapter 8 highlights the United Kingdom–based Randomized Evaluations of Accepted Choices in Treatment trials, underscoring lessons learned and best practices for LST investigators. Chapter 9 highlights the workshop participants' insights into strategies moving forward and summarizes the workshop's concluding discussion, in which many participants suggested potential strategies and priorities for accelerating progress in the uptake of LSTs in the United States.

REFERENCES

Clinicaltrials.gov. 2012. *Study of Technology to Accelerate Research (STAR)*. http://clinical trials.gov/show/NCT01537510 (accessed June 17, 2013).

GISSI (Gruppo Italiano per lo Studio della Sopravvivenza nell'Infarto Miocardico). 2013. *What Is GISSI?* http://www.gissi.org/EngIntro/T_Intro_ENG.php (accessed June 17, 2013).

IOM (Institute of Medicine). 2010a. *Transforming Clinical Research in the United States: Challenges and Opportunities: Workshop Summary*. Washington, DC: The National Academies Press.

IOM. 2010b. *Redesigning the Clinical Effectiveness Research Paradigm: Workshop Summary*. Washington, DC: The National Academies Press.

IOM. 2011. *Learning What Works: Infrastructure Required for Comparative Effectiveness Research: Workshop Summary*. Washington, DC: The National Academies Press.

IOM. 2012a. *Envisioning a Transformed Clinical Trials Enterprise in the United States: Establishing an Agenda for 2020: Workshop Summary*. Washington, DC: The National Academies Press.

IOM. 2012b. *Public Engagement and Clinical Trials: New Models and Disruptive Technologies: Workshop Summary*. Washington, DC: The National Academies Press.

Peto, R., R. Collins, and R. Gray. 1995. Large-scale randomized evidence: large, simple trials and overviews of trials. *Journal of Clinical Epidemiology* 48(1):23–40.

RWJF (Robert Wood Johnson Foundation). 2013. *Health Information Technology in the United States: Better Information Systems for Better Care.* Princeton, NJ: RWJF. http://www.rwjf.org/content/dam/farm/reports/reports/2013/rwjf406758 (accessed June 20, 2013).

Sung, N. S., W. F. Crowley, M. Genel, P. Salber, L. Sandy, L. M. Sherwood, S. B. Johnson, V. Catanese, H. Tilson, K. Getz, E. L. Larson, D. Scheinberg, E. A. Reece, H. Slavkin, A. Dobs, J. Grebb, R. A. Martinez, A. Korn, and D. Rimoin. 2003. Central challenges facing the national clinical research enterprise. *Journal of the American Medical Association* 289(10):1278–1287.

Tufts Center for the Study of Drug Development. 2012. *News Report: Extraneous Data Collected in Clinical Trials Cost Drug Developers $4 Billion to $6 Billion Annually.* http://csdd.tufts.edu/news/complete_story/pr_ir_nov-dec_2012 (accessed June 19, 2013).

2

Large Simple Trials Now
and Looking Forward

KEY SPEAKER THEMES

Lauer

- The promise of large simple trials (LSTs) should not be discounted on the basis of their current limitations. History is riddled with disruptive innovations that displace older, less efficient technologies or approaches.
- LSTs and greater patient involvement in research will be key to moving the health care system to a future in which every clinical encounter is an opportunity for learning.

Horwitz

- LSTs pose a series of challenges and opportunities for the clinical research enterprise. These include solidification of their external validity, a better understanding of the implications of LSTs for the detection of treatment heterogeneity and patient safety, and exploration of opportunities for greater integration of patient-reported outcomes.
- Care must be taken to prevent LSTs from becoming large, complex trials. It will be important to preserve the efficiency of LSTs while their value for clinical decision making by physicians and patients is cemented.

INTRODUCTION

The concept of large simple trials (LSTs) is not new, but the number of LSTs conducted is very small compared with the number of complex and often small clinical trials conducted each year. Although LSTs are uncommon, they have proven the effectiveness of treatments for common diseases, such as the early use of intravenous streptokinase during heart attacks and low-dose aspirin to reduce the risk of a first heart attack. They have also shown that some treatments are not effective, for example, that vitamin E does not prevent cancer.

Michael S. Lauer, director of the Division of Cardiovascular Sciences at the National Heart, Lung, and Blood Institute, part of the National Institutes of Health, described his vision for the future of clinical research in which many simplified trials are carried out in regular care settings, making each clinical encounter an opportunity for learning. Ralph I. Horwitz, senior vice president for clinical sciences evaluation at GlaxoSmithKline, addressed the challenges as well as the opportunities posed by LSTs.

A VISION FOR LARGE SIMPLE TRIALS IN THE LEARNING HEALTH SYSTEM

Michael S. Lauer gave a cautionary talk addressing those who might oppose the use of LSTs because the data routinely collected in electronic health records (EHRs) are inferior in detail and quality to data collected for traditional randomized controlled trials (RCTs). He likened this view to that of Eastman Kodak of the first digital camera images. They were substantially inferior to film images, which made it easy for Kodak to dismiss the importance of digital camera technology.

Lauer thus began his talk by holding up an Instamatic camera, a popular film camera made by Kodak from the 1960s into the 1980s. He pointed to the year 1976, when Steven Sasson, a Kodak engineer, invented the digital camera, which has subsequently proceeded to eclipse the photographic film and film camera business almost completely. Although the technology was developed by Kodak, the company decided not to exploit its advantage and stuck to its film-based business model. After all, Kodak had 85 percent of the camera market and 90 percent of the film market in 1976. Although Kodak eventually produced digital cameras, the effort was too little, too late to halt the company's decline. It filed for Chapter 11 bankruptcy protection in 2012. Lauer told the audience to remember the Kodak Instamatic before dismissing the LST model at its current stage of development.

Kodak's failure to see that a new technology would destroy its business is not a unique case, Lauer noted. It is common for large organizations to have difficulty dealing with innovative technologies because they are successful with their current business model, the new technology is usually initially inferior, and their established customers are not asking for it.

Lauer showed a figure from the work of Clayton Christensen, of Harvard Business School. Christensen coined the term "disruptive innovation" to describe the process in which a new product or service disregarded by established competitors is developed by others, becomes attractive to new customers at the bottom of the market, moves upmarket, and eventually outperforms the established technologies (see Figure 2-1) (Christensen, 1997). Lauer explained that over time, the performance of any given technology increases through incremental improvements made by competitors but eventually plateaus (the red line in Figure 2-1). At some point, the performance of a new technology developed by other organizations exceeds that of the older technology (where the blue line crosses the red line in Figure 2-1), rendering the older technology obsolete (blue and red lines at Time 2 in Figure 2-1).

Lauer then described the standard business model for RCTs, which he likened to the Kodak business model. Most RCTs involve a small number of subjects able to meet a narrow set of criteria and collect large amounts of very specific data on each subject. RCT recruitment and data collection, monitoring, and auditing processes are very costly; and often, RCTs can be supported only in academic medical centers. Moreover, given the relatively small sample sizes that they require, surrogate endpoints rather than clinical

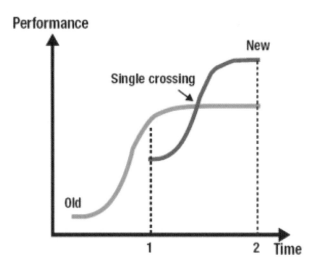

FIGURE 2-1 Pathway of disruptive innovation over time.
SOURCE: Reprinted with permission from Michael S. Lauer.

endpoints, which are often of more interest to patients and the clinicians caring for them, are often used.

What might a new model look like?, Lauer asked. He referred to GISSI (Gruppo Italiano per lo Studio della Sopravvivenza nell'Infarto Miocardico), a very large, very simple clinical trial conducted in Italy in 1984 and 1985 that proved that early thrombolytic treatment with streptokinase on in-hospital mortality of patients with acute myocardial infarction is efficacious (GISSI, 2013). The GISSI trial involved nearly 12,000 patients being treated in 176 coronary care units who were enrolled over 17 months at a cost of 30 euros per patient. Although GISSI was inexpensive and short, its findings had an enormous impact on clinical practice.

Other LSTs have been and are being conducted, although they constitute a small share of all clinical trials. Lauer described the Thrombus Aspiration in ST-Elevation Myocardial Infarction (TASTE) trial, in which 5,000 patients in Scandinavia with acute myocardial infarction are being randomized to percutaneous coronary intervention (PCI), the standard treatment, or to thrombus aspiration followed by PCI. Nearly all the data used for the TASTE trial have already been collected by existing registries. As a result, the trial is large enough to yield a meaningful outcome, yet the cost is very small compared with that of most trials.

Lauer identified greater patient involvement in their health care as another disruptive technology, especially in the area of rare diseases. As an example, he pointed to a trial of the efficacy and safety of sirolimus in lymphangioleiomyomatosis (LAM), a progressive and often fatal cystic lung disease primarily affecting women. It was possible to conduct a trial for a disease that affects only 5 in 1 million women because a significant number of LAM patients were willing to participate in clinical trials through their organization, the LAM Foundation, to which many had already contributed clinical profiles.

Lauer proposed a new model that integrates trials into routine clinical care and that would involve the simultaneous conduct of many LSTs. They would enroll huge numbers of patients, which would enable robust estimates of treatment effects even among subgroups. However, the costs would be small because the research designs would be simple and existing data sources would be used. They would take place in general medical settings. The endpoints would be patient oriented with minimal or no adjudication. Theoretically, every patient could be enrolled in a clinical trial unless the patient has a disease that is already curable. Such LSTs would be an integral part of the learning health care system, because every clinical encounter would include an invitation to participate in a new clinical trial or a follow-up of an ongoing clinical trial.

OPPORTUNITIES AND CHALLENGES FOR LSTs

In his presentation, Ralph I. Horwitz laid out for the workshop participants the opportunities that LSTs could provide to improve clinical decision making by providers and by patients and the challenges to achieving this without turning LSTs into large complex trials. He posited that modern information technologies, such EHRs, could be harnessed to provide more detailed clinical data for LSTs without reducing the efficiencies of those LSTs.

He began by reviewing the case for LSTs, stating that trials of promising treatments with important but small to moderate treatment effects must have a very large number of participants to detect an effect with certainty. Because differences in the direction of treatment effects (positive or negative) are quite uncommon and differences in the magnitudes of treatment effects are likely to be equally distributed between groups, enrollment in an LST can be simple and therefore fast and cheap. Also, as LSTs are conducted in general medical settings with busy clinicians, the interventions need to be simple, which also means that they are more likely to achieve widespread adoption if they prove to be successful.

Horwitz said it was important to talk about what he called the "challentunities"—that is, the challenges and the opportunities—posed by LSTs. He identified four areas of "challentunities":

1. Verification of the external validity of LSTs,
2. Treatment heterogeneity,
3. Patient safety, and
4. Patient-reported outcomes (PROs).

External Validity

LSTs, Horwitz said, are generally considered to have greater external validity than small RCTs with strict entry criteria, and therefore, their results are expected to be more applicable to the general patient population. A potential strength of LSTs compared with RCTs is their ability to detect small treatment effects that could confer substantial benefit when applied to an entire population. Therefore, the results of LSTs, even when they are strongly positive, are likely to have small impacts on individual patients.

Horwitz asked if it is possible that a very small benefit shown by an LST might have a negative benefit in the intended target population. He noted that LSTs, like all clinical trials, have selection criteria, and therefore, it is possible that patients meeting those criteria may have a response different from that of the overall target population. For example, he said, in the GISSI trial cited by Michael S. Lauer, only 45 percent of the 43,000 patients admitted to the coronary care units of the participating hospitals were randomized in the trial. The others had clinical characteristics that made them ineligible. Because the absolute risk reduction shown by the GISSI intervention was just 1.4 percent and the mortality rate of the excluded patients was quite different (about double), it is possible that the intervention might have a negative effect on the general population that was not detected in the trial.

Horwitz suggested that the proponents of LSTs need to address whether the application of the results of LSTs to the entire target population will, in fact, achieve the benefits observed in the design of the original study. It is not a reason not to do these trials, he said, but it is a reason to think hard about the effects on individual patients and whether the net benefit for the population is that which is intended.

Treatment Heterogeneity

Treatment heterogeneity refers to the different degrees of impact that an intervention might have on subgroups within the population, such as those with certain comorbid conditions. An assumption made in LSTs, Horwitz said, is that treatment heterogeneity is unlikely to be a major problem. Although effects may differ between subgroups, they are likely to be in the same direction (positive or negative) and not qualitatively different enough to be of practical concern. This allows LSTs to avoid collecting detailed information on each participant, an important advantage in terms of the cost and the complexity of conducting LSTs.

However, an understanding of treatment heterogeneity can be very valuable in clinical trials. Horwitz asked if it is possible to validly and efficiently look at treatment heterogeneity by collecting the relevant clinical and laboratory data within an LST. He predicted that a recurring topic of the workshop would be the extent to which EHRs, as they are currently constituted, could provide data for subgroup analyses easily and cheaply and how the future development of EHRs could better enable this.

Patient Safety

Horwitz asserted that ensuring the safety as well as the effectiveness of medicines is a fundamental, critical requirement in the preapproval period for all new medicines and increasingly in the postapproval period. Well-tested procedures for assessing the safety risk in new medicines exist. When adverse events occur with any new medicine, detailed data on the clinical context in which the adverse event occurred are required for regulatory review and approval. Horwitz noted that it can be frustrating to rely on data collected for other purposes to identify the antecedent events associated with an adverse event when the relevant data were not systematically collected as part of the original data collection process. He noted that it will be important to determine how to suitably assess the safety of medicines and devices through streamlined approaches such as LSTs, if they are to be used for those purposes.

Patient-Reported Outcomes

PROs, such as measures of morbidity or quality of life, are becoming an important part of clinical trials, but they are not well captured by the usual standardized measures used in RCTs. Horwitz suggested that LSTs might be an opportunity to better incorporate PROs into systematic assessments, expanding the value of LSTs for patients and physicians. He was optimistic that new information technologies will assist with the collection of data from and about patients without reductions in the efficiencies of LSTs.

Conclusion

Horwitz concluded by warning against turning LSTs into large complex trials. The question before the workshop participants, he continued, was how to preserve the efficiency of those trials while increasing their value for clinical decision making by physicians and patients. He noted that one way will be to use information technology to design and conduct LSTs. They can then be conducted without requiring patients to travel to brick-and-mortar research facilities by using electronic information technology systems for recruitment, informed consent, medication orders, and follow-up. Horwitz mentioned that a group called Mytrus is trying to pioneer such approaches and that social media like PatientsLikeMe could be used to obtain PROs.

REFERENCES

Christensen, C. 1997. *The Innovator's Dilemma: When New Technologies Cause Great Firms to Fail.* Boston, MA: Harvard Business School Press.

GISSI (Gruppo Italiano per lo Studio della Sopravvivenza nell'Infarto Miocardico). 2013. *What Is GISSI?* http://www.gissi.org/EngIntro/T_Intro_ENG.php (accessed June 17, 2013).

3

Examples of Large Simple Trials

KEY SPEAKER THEMES

Manson

- The VITamin D and omegA 3 triaL (VITAL) is an example of a two-by-two factorial, placebo-controlled prevention trial being done primarily through the mail with a very large, demographically representative cohort.
- VITAL has a cost-efficient hybrid design involving ascertainment of incident clinical events in 25,000 participants nationwide, together with in-clinic visits and in-depth phenotyping of a subset of 1,000 participants.

Choudhry

- The Myocardial Infarction Free Rx (Prescription) Event and Economic Evaluation (MI FREEE) trial was done in partnership with a payer to test whether the elimination of out-of-pocket expenses for medications taken after a myocardial infarction would improve patient adherence to prescription medications and clinical outcomes.
- The MI FREEE trial demonstrated that it is possible to conduct large simple trials (LSTs) with clinical and policy relevance.

Taveras

- The High Five for Kids and Study of Technology to Accelerate Research (STAR) trials are electronic health record (EHR)-based LSTs done to test antiobesity interventions in pediatric populations.
- EHR systems can be very useful for identification of potential trial participants, data collection, and provision of decision support tools for parents and clinicians.

Devereaux

- The Heart Outcomes Prevention Evaluation (HOPE) trial was a large, randomized trial of the angiotensin-converting-enzyme inhibitor ramipril and vitamin E in patients at high risk of cardiovascular events.
- Consideration of the applicability of the results during the trial design led to a widespread impact on clinician practice.

INTRODUCTION

The part of the workshop described in this chapter was devoted to presentations describing four large simple trials (LSTs), some ongoing and some completed, that have different features of interest. JoAnn E. Manson, chief of the Division of Preventive Medicine at Brigham and Women's Hospital and the Michael and Lee Bell Professor of Women's Health at Harvard Medical School, presented an overview of the ongoing VITamin D and omegA 3 triaL (VITAL). Niteesh K. Choudhry, Department of Medicine, Brigham and Women's Hospital, and associate professor, Harvard Medical School, reviewed the Post-Myocardial Infarction Free Rx (Prescription) Event and Economic Evaluation (MI FREEE) Trial. Elsie M. Taveras, associate professor of population medicine, Harvard Pilgrim Health Care Institute, Harvard Medical School, reviewed two LSTs, High Five for Kids and the Study of Technology to Accelerate Research (STAR). P. J. Devereaux, Population Health Research Institute, McMaster University, discussed the Heart Outcomes Prevention Evaluation (HOPE) study.

VITAMIN D AND OMEGA 3 TRIAL

The VITamin D and omegA 3 triaL (VITAL; http://www.vitalstudy.org) is an example of an ongoing, placebo-controlled, primary prevention LST testing the efficacy of nutritional interventions in preventing cardiovascular disease (CVD) and cancer and is sponsored by the National Institutes of Health (NIH). The trial is assessing whether daily vitamin D_3 or omega 3 fatty acid supplements, or both (in a two-by-two factorial design), reduces the risk of heart disease, stroke, or cancer in people with no history of those diseases.

Manson began her presentation by responding to a discussion that took place after earlier presentations about the feasibility of conducting blinded placebo-controlled LSTs with large number of participants in scattered locations. She noted that large simple placebo-controlled trials had been successfully conducted by mail even before the advent of the Internet, citing the Physicians' Health Study, which delivered study pills in foil-backed calendar (blister) packs by mail. She commented that it was not clear why this approach had not been adopted more widely, especially with the availability of mobile devices to stay in contact with participants. In her view, many opportunities to conduct LSTs exist.

Manson discussed several completed placebo-controlled LSTs that yielded important answers about potentially effective interventions at very low cost—between $100 and $200 in direct costs per participant per year. The first Physicians' Health Study, for example, enrolled more than 22,000 physicians and showed that aspirin substantially reduced the risk of a first heart attack. Although the Women's Health Study found that aspirin caused a significant reduction in the incidence of stroke in women, vitamin E was found to have a null effect on the incidence of both CVD and cancer. Another study, the Women's Antioxidant and Folic Acid Study, found no evidence of a benefit or harm of beta-carotene, vitamins C and E, folic acid, and vitamins B_6, B_{12}, C, and E on the incidence of CVD events or cancer. These trials' findings have been concordant with the results of other trials with much higher costs per participant.

Manson noted that the studies mentioned above were conducted with health professional populations to facilitate the collection of informed consent and to ensure high rates of compliance with the consumption of the medications as directed, high response rates to questionnaires, and approval for medical record review. What is different about VITAL, she said, is that it is being conducted with a population that is sociodemographically representative of the U.S. population and not just health care professionals. The purpose of VITAL is to conclusively determine whether two promising interventions—vitamin D_3 and omega 3 fatty acids from fish—reduce the risk of cancer or CVD, or both.

VITAL has enrolled 25,000 healthy older individuals (men age 50 years and older, women age 55 years and older), which will give the trial sufficient statistical power to detect 10 to 15 percent reductions in the primary outcomes. Participants are being randomly assigned to one of four treatment groups: vitamin D_3 (2,000 international units a day) and placebo, omega 3 (1 gram per day) and placebo, both vitamin D_3 and omega 3, or two placebos. VITAL is a 5-year double-blind trial in which the pills are being provided by mail in blister packs without the participants or their providers knowing if the pills contain active ingredients or placebo.

The entry criteria for VITAL include few criteria for exclusion in an effort to recruit participants representative of the general population. The trial has made a special effort to recruit members of racial and ethnic minority groups to ensure diversity and is on track to achieve its demographic goals. Manson detailed how 16,000 participants will provide initial blood samples and 6,000 will provide follow-up blood samples. The trial also has a hybrid design involving in-clinic visits for a subset of participants. In the Boston, Massachusetts, area, 1,000 participants are having in-depth and extensive clinical assessments (anthropometrics, blood pressure, 2-hour oral glucose tolerance tests, physical performance assessments, and imaging studies) at the baseline and after 2 years. These evaluations will enable a number of ancillary studies.

POST-MYOCARDIAL INFARCTION FREE RX EVENT AND ECONOMIC EVALUATION TRIAL

Within 2 years, up to half of the patients who have suffered a heart attack, or acute myocardial infarction (MI), stop taking evidence-based primary prevention therapies—such as aspirin, beta-blockers, angiotensin-converting-enzyme (ACE) inhibitors, angiotensin receptor blockers (ARBs), and statins—to reduce the risk of another cardiovascular event. Some observational evidence indicates that the out-of-pocket costs of medications prescribed after a heart attack are a major factor in the high degree of nonadherence to doctors' orders. To determine whether this is the case, the MI FREEE trial tested whether elimination of out-of-pocket expenses for medications prescribed after an MI would increase the percentage of patients who continue to take their medications as prescribed and therefore improve clinical outcomes and was described by Niteesh K. Chuoudhry (Choudhry, 2011). The outcomes measured were the rate of readmissions for fatal and nonfatal MI; the incidence of unstable angina, heart failure, and stroke; and the need for coronary revascularization. The trial was funded by Aetna and the Commonwealth Foundation.

Chuoudhry noted that the MI FREEE trial was able to be large and simple by the use of electronic health insurance claims to collect most of the data. Six thousand participants were identified through a search of Aetna beneficiary records for those recently discharged from the hospital after an MI, and the participants were followed for 1 year. Patients who agreed to participate were randomized into two groups. The intervention, or full-coverage, group was informed that their pharmacies would not charge them for their post-MI medications, whereas members of the control group received their usual coverage for prescriptions. Patients in the trial were contacted only once, Choudhry emphasized. The information on prescriptions filled, clinical outcomes, and costs was extracted from claims and the National Death Index through the use of health services research techniques.

Choudhry reported that the study did not find significant differences between the full-coverage and usual-coverage groups in the primary outcome, a major vascular event, or the need for revascularization. However, it did find significant differences in outcomes for the secondary endpoints. For example, although the adherence rates were just 41 to 55 percent in the full-coverage group, those rates were 4 to 6 percentage points higher than those for the usual-coverage group, a significant difference. The rate of major vascular events among patients in the full-coverage group was 14 percent less than that among patients in the usual-coverage group, a statistically and clinically significant difference. On average, patient spending was less in the full-coverage than the usual-coverage group ($526 and $900, respectively) without increasing overall costs ($18,254 and $20,238, respectively).

Choudhry mentioned some limitations of the study, such as the lag time between the initial MI and randomization (49 days, on average), the high turnover rate of the insured, and the number of patients who declined to participate; but he concluded that the MI FREEE trial demonstrated that it is possible to conduct LSTs with clinical and policy relevance. He noted that, as a result of the study, Aetna was going to begin reducing copayments for post-MI secondary prevention medications in January 2013.

HIGH FIVE FOR KIDS TRIAL AND STUDY OF TECHNOLOGY TO ACCELERATE RESEARCH

Elsie M. Taveras presented examples of two pediatric LSTs that used electronic health record (EHR) systems for identification of potential participants, data collection, and provision of decision support tools for parents and clinicians.

High Five for Kids was an NIH-funded trial examining whether evidence-based interventions to reduce obesity in children ages 2 through 6 years are effective in a primary care setting rather than a research setting (Taveras, 2011). The High Five for Kids trial involved 500 children seen at 10 pediatric primary care offices who were randomized to usual care or the tested intervention. The intervention included four clinic visits and three motivational telephone calls made by nurse practitioners aimed at reducing television time and the intake of fast food and sugar-sweetened beverages during a 1-year intervention period. Taveras reported that the High Five for Kids trial showed that, after 1 year, the intervention group watched less television and consumed less fast food and sugary drinks than the usual-care group but did not have a significantly lower body mass index (BMI).

She noted that the trial was simplified and able to enroll a large number of children by using the health system's EHR system to identify potential recipients meeting certain BMI criteria. Taveras said that the EHR system was also used to document the completed clinic visits and motivational calls and to assist clinicians with decision support, patient tracking, scheduling, and follow-up. Additionally, the parents in the intervention group were interviewed to obtain demographic information and information about the steps that they took to limit television, fast food, and soft drinks.

The STAR trial (http://clinicaltrials.gov/show/NCT01537510), funded by the Office of Planning and Evaluation of the U.S. Department Health and Human Services, is testing whether health information technology can increase the adoption of evidence-based interventions by parents and clinicians. Specifically, Taveras noted, STAR is seeing if point-of-care alerts and decision support tools in EHRs, with or without direct support and coaching of parents, can increase the adoption of evidence-based approaches to reduce obesity among 6- to 12-year-old children. The trial involves 800 patients at 14 pediatric primary care offices who will be followed for 1 year. The purpose of the trial is to see if the interventions result in increased screening and assessment of childhood obesity, increased counseling on nutrition and physical activity, a smaller increase in BMI, and improved dietary and physical activity behaviors.

As in the High Five for Kids trial, the EHR system is being leveraged to simplify recruitment and to provide best practice alerts and decision support tools to guide clinicians with evidence-based recommendations for patient management, instructions on how to follow up with that patient, what referrals to make, and what patient instructions to print. Taveras noted that the study is also using electronic patient portals for communication between health educators and the families and patients. Finally, the EHR system is being used to obtain point-of-care outcomes, such as Healthcare Effectiveness Data and Information Set (HEDIS) codes; International Classification of Diseases, Ninth Revision, diagnosis codes; and clinical measures of BMI.

HEART OUTCOMES PREVENTION EVALUATION TRIAL

P. J. Devereaux described the HOPE trial, which was funded by the Canadian Institute of Health Research, the Heart and Stroke Foundation of Ontario, Canada, and several drug companies to examine the effects of ramipril versus those of placebo and the effects of vitamin E versus those of placebo on a primary composite endpoint of cardiovascular death, nonfatal

MI, and nonfatal stroke (Heart Outcomes Prevention Evaluation Study Investigators, 2000).

Devereaux described that the HOPE trial was designed to detect a relative risk reduction of 12 percent, which required more than 9,500 patients to be followed for between 4 and 6 years. The criteria for participation were very simple and easy to implement, which was important because the trial included 267 centers in 19 countries. Criteria for recruitment included the following: the participants had to be age 55 years or older; have coronary artery disease, peripheral vascular disease, or stroke or have diabetes and a risk factor for coronary artery disease; and not have heart failure or a low left ventricular ejection fraction and not taking an ACE inhibitor or vitamin E. The HOPE trial found a highly statistically significant reduction in the primary endpoint—the composite of cardiovascular death, non-fatal MI, and stroke—and for each of the individual components of the composite endpoint with the use of ramipril compared with the reduction achieved with the use of placebo.

Devereaux explained that the HOPE trial was designed as an LST because the intent was to see if a treatment would have a relatively modest but highly significant effect on the incidence on a common major health condition that, if successful, would be easy for physicians to apply in clinical practice. This required a large sample size, broad and simple eligibility criteria, a simple intervention that would be easy to implement in real-world clinical settings (one pill a day), and easy data collection. It was also relatively inexpensive, costing $21 million to test two drugs with more than 9,500 patients over 5 years of follow-up, on average. Devereaux reported that the positive effect of ramipril was quickly evident and the trial was terminated early. The impact on clinician practice was also quick because the result—by design—was widely applicable.

REFERENCES

Choudhry, N., J. Avorn, R. J. Glynn, E. M. Antman, S. Schneeweiss, M. Toscano, L. Reisman, J. Fernandes, C. Spettell, J. L. Lee, R. Levin, T. Brennan, W. H. Shrank, and the Post-Myocardial Infarction Free Rx Event and Economic Evaluation (MI FREEE) Trial. 2011. Full coverage for preventative medications after myocardial infarction. *New England Journal of Medicine* 365:2088–2097.

Heart Outcomes Prevention Evaluation Study Investigators. 2000. Effects of an angiotensin-converting-enzyme inhibitor, ramipril on cardiovascular events in high-risk patients. *New England Journal of Medicine* 342(3):145–153.

Taveras, E. M., S. L. Gortmaker, K. H. Hohman, C. M. Horan, K. P. Kleinman, K. Mitchell, S. Price, L. A. Prosser, S. L. Rifas-Shiman, and M. W. Gillman. 2011. Randomized controlled trial to improve primary care to prevent and manage childhood obesity. *Archives of Pediatrics & Adolescent Medicine* 165(8):714–722.

4

Medical Product Regulatory Issues

┌───┐

KEY SPEAKER THEMES

Getz

- A variety of factors contribute to the complexity of clinical trials, including a shift in focus from acute to chronic illness, collection of increasingly intricate data elements, and concern about potential requests from regulatory agencies.
- Trial complexity not only increases direct study costs but also negatively affects broad-level trial performance.
- Closer attention to each element in the trial design could help to alleviate the complexity associated with unnecessary procedures, protocol amendments, and irrelevant data collection.

Granger

- Trial quality is driven by whether it answers an important question that will change clinical practice and improve outcomes.
- Opportunities exist to reduce the costs of clinical trials without compromising quality through the use of a variety of simplification approaches, either incremental or transformative.
- The reasons that many of these cost-saving strategies have not been more widely implemented may have to do with investiga-

└───┘

tor and sponsor risk aversion, interest in maintaining the status quo, and a lack of international harmonization.

Sherman

- The U.S. Food and Drug Administration (FDA) does not emphasize a particular trial design in its regulations; instead, it emphasizes the quality of the clinical data produced.
- FDA's primary concerns are the safety of the patient and the quality of the data from the clinical trial.
- Consulting early and often with FDA on trial design and the primary endpoints offers the promise to ensure a well-designed, productive study.

INTRODUCTION

Clinical trials of all designs, including large simple trials, are often overly complex and costly. This chapter summarizes panel discussions on the current state of trial complexity, various strategies for reducing the complexity of clinical trials and increasing their efficacy, and the U.S. Food and Drug Administration's (FDA's) perspective on clinical trial design. Kenneth A. Getz, director of sponsored research programs and research associate professor at the Tufts Center for the Study of Drug Development, discussed the mounting complexity of today's clinical trials and highlighted possible reasons for the prevalence of such complexity. Christopher B. Granger, director of the Duke University Cardiac Care Unit and professor of medicine at the Duke University Medical Center, continued the panel discussions with a presentation on the promise offered by simplification strategies for reducing the costs of clinical trials and increasing their effectiveness. Rachel E. Sherman, associate director of medical policy for the Center for Drug Evaluation and Research at FDA, brought the panel to a close with a discussion of FDA's perspective on clinical trial design.

TRIAL COMPLEXITY

In his discussion of complexity in current clinical trial protocols, Kenneth A. Getz underscored the increasing number of elements measured and incorporated into clinical trials today. A typical study has an average of 13 endpoints: 1 primary endpoint, 5 key secondary endpoints, and a number of tertiary, or exploratory, endpoints. Moreover, the average study protocol involves nearly 170 procedures, only half of which support the primary and key secondary endpoints. The typical protocol also has an av-

TABLE 4-1 Rising Protocol Complexity and Burden

	00–03	04–07	08–11
Unique procedures per protocol (median)	20.5	28.2	30.4
Total procedures per protocol (median)	105.9	158.1	166.6
Total investigative site work burden (median units)	28.9	44.6	47.5
Total eligibility criteria	31	38	35
Median number of CRF pages per protocol	55	180	169

NOTE: CRF = case report form.
SOURCE: Reprinted with permission from Kenneth A. Getz.

erage of 35 eligibility criteria, and the case report form for a typical clinical trial has nearly 170 pages, requiring a study volunteer to make 11 visits over an average of 175 days of participation in a trial. Additionally, Getz emphasized, as studies are simultaneously conducted in a growing number of countries, the requisite coordination with multiple health authorities and different regulatory agencies and the logistics of distributing clinical supplies and collecting data in ever more remote regions add large amounts of complexity. Table 4-1 documents these items over the course of three observation periods in the past 10 years. Getz explained that each element has experienced a significant increase, contributing to the rising complexity and burden of clinical trial protocols.

To explain this increase, Getz continued, one could look to the shift in focus from acute illness to chronic illness, for which endpoints are far more difficult to measure. Moreover, many current studies are collecting more genetic material and biomarker data and involve a combination treatment or a diagnostic procedure, both of which add complexity and additional procedures to the clinical trial protocol. More data are being collected at all phases of clinical trials, Getz said, possibly because of pressure from regulatory agencies to collect more safety data or to determine whether a project should be terminated early. Particularly during Phase III trials, more data are collected in anticipation of regulatory requests, and even Phase IV studies have shifted from being more observational in nature to more robust, controlled clinical trials.

This continuously increasing complexity negatively affects the performance of clinical trials in a variety of ways, Getz explained. More complex trials have worse recruitment and retention rates and also have prolonged cycle times. Additionally, more complex trials typically correlate with more amendments to the trial design, which can be incredibly costly and disruptive to implement. Research has shown that the majority of protocols have at least one amendment, 46 percent of which occur before the first patient receives the first dose. Nearly 40 percent of all amendments are deemed avoidable by those companies sponsoring the studies. Getz cited inappropriate or irrelevant policies, typographical errors, and design flaws as potential reasons for these amendments, underscoring the idea that a protocol amendment is not a problem; it is instead a solution to an underlying design problem. However, one such solution typically adds roughly 2 months to the overall length of a study and costs about half a million dollars in direct study costs.

Getz ended with a discussion of the following question: is all of this complexity meaningful? In a study of companies sponsoring clinical trials and their specific protocols, almost one out every five protocols was classified by the protocol designers to be noncore in nature: the protocol was not tied to a primary or key secondary endpoint, it was not associated with good clinical practice compliance, and it was not evaluating a procedure typically performed in the clinical setting. Possible reasons for such a high proportion of noncore procedures, Getz elaborated, include a desire to collect additional data to gain insight into a particular mechanism of action of a drug or even a new area of development, along with efforts to mitigate the risk that regulatory agencies will request additional data or resistance by purchasers and payers to pay for the drug once it is approved and on the market. Additionally, protocol designs from earlier phases of clinical trials are often reused for later studies, without consideration of whether all procedures from the former studies are necessary for the latter ones.

As a final point of measurement, Getz highlighted that roughly 18 cents of every dollar that is spent on clinical trials goes toward these noncore, or less essential, procedures. This approaches $2 million per Phase III study budget, or $4 billion to $6 billion per year worldwide. Further scrutiny of trial elements and procedures, Getz concluded, would assist with simplification of protocol designs and could not only alleviate some of these misdirected costs but also improve trial performance.

SIMPLIFYING CLINICAL TRIALS

Christopher B. Granger began his remarks by underscoring several key points: trial quality can be defined, large simple trials can be burdened with complexity that does not improve quality, examples of trials that are much simpler and fit for their purpose exist, trials could be either radically or incrementally simplified in most circumstances, and cost reductions resulting from sensible simplification can be quantified. He continued by indicating that trial quality is driven by an important question that will change practice and improve outcomes. With this understanding, Granger elaborated, trial quality is determined by a number of elements, including the availability of an adequate number of events to answer the research question with confidence, proper randomization, and a plan for ongoing measurement and feedback for improvement of quality measures during the conduct of the trial (see Box 4-1).

Granger delved into the question of how to reduce not only the costs of clinical trials but also their complexity. Using a hypothetical trial of a treatment for a chronic disease with 20,000 patients across 1,000 sites performed over 2 years with 60 case report form pages, 24 site visits, and a study award of $10,000 per patient, researchers prepared models for three different cost estimates: a model of the cost of the full trial, a model of the cost of a streamlined trial, and a model of the cost of a radically streamlined trial. The model of the cost of the full trial provided a cost of roughly $400 million.

To calculate the cost of a streamlined trial, a variety of factors were altered. The trial duration, trial size (in terms of the length of the case report form and the number of sites), and operational issues were all adjusted. Of particular importance was accounting for the large number of unproductive trial sites. Granger described the work of Lisa Berdan and the Duke Clinical Research Institute showing that the top 10 percent of trial sites enroll about 40 percent of all patients. Moreover, the cost of starting up the trial at each site is significant, estimated to be a minimum of $14,000, so the removal of those sites that will not be productive is a critical source

---

BOX 4-1
Elements Determining the Quality of a Clinical Trial

The trial must be performed

- with an adequate number of events to answer the question with confidence;
- in a practice setting to make results generalizable;
- with proper randomization;
- with reasonably complete follow-up and definitive ascertainment of the primary outcome;
- with an aggregate safety assessment;
- with a plan for ongoing measurement, feedback, and improvement of quality measures during the conduct of the trial;
- with safeguards against bias in determining clinically relevant outcomes (like blinding); and
- with protection of the rights of the participants.

SOURCE: Reprinted with permission from Christopher B. Granger.

of preventable expense. Reductions in the amount of time for planning and enrollment resulted in relatively modest cost reductions, with only a 1 to 2 percent reduction in the total cost of the trial. However, Granger explained that decreases in the length of the case report form and the number of sites had much more significant impacts, with a nearly 10 percent reduction in cost being obtained after a modest reduction in the total number of sites. Electronic data capture offered the potential for a 10 percent reduction in cost through the elimination of query processing, data entry, and medical coding; and it also decreased the amount of time required for management of queries. Lastly, adjustment of site management factors, including streamlining of trial procedures and reduction of the number of physician visits to the study site, decreased costs by 21 percent. Granger reported that the changes made in the model of a streamlined trial yielded a 35 percent reduction in costs. Additionally, further extension of these changes to include a 50 percent lower per patient study award reduced costs by a dramatic 60 percent.

The model of the cost of a radically streamlined trial, which was limited to 100 high-volume sites, eliminated on-site evaluations and source data verification, used highly focused case report forms, and dramatically reduced payments to the study sites. With this model, the cost of the trial was reduced nearly 10-fold from the cost for the full study.

Granger continued his discussion of approaches to streamlined trial design by highlighting the Thrombus Aspiration in ST-Elevation Myocardial Infarction (TASTE) trial in Sweden as a case study (Fröbert et al., 2010). Built on the Swedish acute myocardial infarction (MI) registry, this trial randomly assigned patients with acute MI to thrombus aspiration with primary percutaneous coronary intervention (PCI) or primary PCI alone. With the registry, researchers were able to identify and register eligible patients, record whether those patients had provided verbal informed consent, and confirm that the inclusion/exclusion criteria had been met. The incremental cost of these procedures has been about $50 per patient, or $350,000 for all 7,000 participants.

To conclude, Granger asked why these cost-reducing strategies have not been adopted, as they have already proven effective. Aversion to the risk of having not collected a particular element requested by auditors is one possible explanation; researchers may believe that it is better to collect 100 unnecessary variables than to miss one important one. Additionally, Granger explained, regulatory departments and contract research organizations have a substantial financial stake in maintaining the status quo, as their business models and margins are created by the complexity inherent to current trial designs. Lastly, the lack of international harmonization among trial designs can force the use of the most complicated common denominator.

Granger underscored the fact that each trial is different, and thus, no universal solutions for simplification exist. However, substantial reductions in the costs of large-scale clinical trials can be achieved without compromising quality, and these savings can be achieved through both incremental and transformational simplification approaches. Further research on the impact of the simplification of clinical trials will help to transition the current research paradigm to one that is more effective and efficient.

FDA PERSPECTIVE

Rachel E. Sherman concluded the panel's discussions by sharing the FDA's perspective and providing guidance on the design of clinical trials. She began her comments with an emphasis on the need for researchers and sponsors to work with FDA more regularly throughout the research process. Moreover, she underscored that unproductive trials, those trials that do not produce useful insights, not only are wasteful but also are unethical for the research enterprise. With the resources available in the United States and around the world, Sherman stressed, it should be possible to address the existing evidence gap in medical research, but continued that wasteful protocols and procedures hinder progress.

Sherman continued by underscoring the idea that the collection of extraneous data points attributed to a fear of regulatory agencies is not supported by the reality of FDA's regulatory practices; what truly matters is meeting the primary endpoint. Of the utmost importance to FDA is data quality, Sherman explained, and only high-quality data can provide substantial evidence. Substantial evidence, as defined by the Food Drug and Cosmetic (FD&C) Act, is "evidence consisting of adequate and well-controlled investigations, including clinical investigations, by experts qualified by scientific training and experience, to evaluate the effectiveness of the drug involved, on the basis of which it can be fairly and responsibly concluded by such experts that the drug will have the effect it purports or is represented to have under the conditions of use prescribed, recommended, or suggested in the labeling and proposed labeling thereof" (Section 505(d) of the FD&C Act).

The FD&C Act, Sherman emphasized, does not prescribe a particular trial design but instead states that the trial must produce evidence, be appropriately designed, and produce useful information. It is then the responsibility of FDA to communicate that information. As such, large simple trials are not discouraged by FDA but instead only need to adhere to the parameters set forth by FDA's bylaws. Again, FDA's emphasis is not on the specific design of a trial but on the quality of the data that it produces.

Moreover, concerns about FDA's directive to come and inspect well-designed, controlled, and adequate trials are unwarranted, Sherman said. FDA has the authority to put on hold any trial that is not adequate and well controlled, as well as any Phase II or Phase III study whose design is clearly deficient in its ability to meet the stated objectives of the study. Most importantly, if the trial presents an unreasonable risk to a patient, FDA of course has the regulatory authority to put it on hold; the patient must always come first, Sherman emphasized. If these characteristics do not apply to the trial in question, concerns about FDA inspection or requests for additional data points may be unnecessary.

In terms of harmonization, Sherman continued, FDA has been focused on the streamlining of clinical trials to modernize and harmonize trial design. The goal is to collect only those data needed and to monitor only the necessary procedures. Again, early discussions with FDA can help to ensure that the right questions are being asked and can assuage later fears of FDA monitoring or requests for additional data.

Sherman closed by underscoring that FDA does not emphasize a particular type of trial; the agency instead emphasizes the collection of high-quality data and not a large quantity of data, and once a trial is completed, it will confirm the quality and generalizability of those data. She requested that workshop attendees communicate with the agency if they believe that it is not promoting the use of more efficient designs to ensure that FDA is doing its part to continue the conversation and advance the field.

REFERENCES

Fröbert, O., B. Lagerqvist, T. Gudnason, L. Thuesen, R. Svennson, G. K. Olivecrona, and S. K. James. 2010. Thrombus Aspiration in ST-Elevation Myocardial Infarction in Scandinavia (TASTE trial). *American Heart Journal* 160(6):1042–1048.

Getz, K. A., R. A. Campo, and K. I. Kaitin. 2011. Variability in protocol design complexity by phase and therapeutic area. *Drug Information Journal* 45(4):413–420.

5

Infrastructure Needs and Opportunities

KEY SPEAKER THEMES

Platt

- Large simple trials (LSTs) should make every attempt to not interfere with the normal work flow of a clinical operation.
- Electronic health records (EHRs) are useful and possibly essential for obtaining the benefits of LSTs but are not a panacea.
- Organizational consortia, often required to conduct LSTs, are expensive and have complicated governance challenges.

Ferguson

- It is possible to do an LST at the point of care.
- The questions being asked by LSTs should be driven by the information needs of clinical practice.
- The greater use of LSTs will require a rethinking of the relationship between research and clinical care.

Kush

- Technologies and resources that would allow the conduct of regulated clinical research from electronic sources, in particular, EHRs, without the use of paper exist.

- The use of these approaches could lead to great advances in research efficiency, quality, and cost. They are particularly suited to use with LSTs.
- Given the maturity of these resources, guidance from the U.S. Food and Drug Administration, and the support of vendors, the only thing missing is a sponsor willing to be the first to conduct a trial with data from an EHR.

Lannon

- Reusable networks can be a way to engage patients, families, clinicians, and researchers and for clinicians and institutions to learn from a patient population much larger than the one that they serve.
- These networks can effectively use technologies to collect data once and serve many purposes, including population management, quality reporting, and research.
- Advances in information technology hold much promise for the future of data networks that pull data from many diverse sources.

INTRODUCTION

Large simple trials (LSTs) are attractive because they can answer certain questions about the effectiveness of drugs and other interventions at less cost or in less time, or both, than the standard randomized clinical trial (RCT). In this session of the workshop, presenters addressed the infrastructure needs for the greater adoption of LSTs and the opportunities for and benefits of relying on electronic health records (EHRs) and other information systems and organizational arrangements to conduct LSTs.

Richard Platt, professor and chair of the Harvard Medical School Department of Population Medicine at the Harvard Pilgrim Health Care Institute, addressed the issue of aligning care and research for greater integration. Ryan E. Ferguson, acting director of the U.S. Department of Veterans Affairs (VA) Cooperative Studies Program Coordinating Center in the VA Boston Healthcare System and program director of VA's Point of Care Research Institute shared VA's experiences with carrying out trials with EHR platforms at the point of care. Rebecca Daniels Kush, president and chief executive officer of the Clinical Data Interchange Standards Consortium, discussed opportunities to get research-quality data from EHRs to greatly improve the efficiency of clinical trials. Carole M. Lannon, director of the Learning Networks Core within the James Anderson Center for Health Systems Excellence at Cincinnati Children's Hospital Medical Center and professor of pediatrics at the University of Cincinnati, shared her experiences with building and maintaining reusable research networks.

ALIGNING CARE AND RESEARCH TO REDUCE BURDENS AND IMPROVE INTEGRATION

Richard Platt focused his presentation on three points that resonated with him from earlier sessions of the workshop. First, he noted that LSTs should not interfere with the normal work flow of a clinical operation. Second, he echoed the observation that EHRs are useful and possibly essential for obtaining the benefits of LSTs. Finally, he drew from his own experiences and those of other presenters to state that organizational consortia are often required to conduct LSTs.

LSTs Should Not Interfere with Normal Clinical Work Flow

Platt noted that, by definition, a clinical trial, even an LST, involves a change in the way in which things are usually done and necessarily affects normal clinical operations. Engagement of the leadership of the health care system involved in the trial is therefore crucial to the success of research done at the point of care, as investment of managerial time and systems support are needed to minimize the impact of a trial on frontline health care providers. Getting support from frontline clinicians can be further facilitated, he suggested, if the trial is testing something that is of interest to them and that can be helpful to their work.

Platt offered the example of a recent LST that he and his colleagues conducted involving 75,000 patients in 43 hospitals of the Hospital Corporation of America (HCA). Although the trial required only minor modifications to regular care, it required significant time and effort from a wide range of other HCA employees, including the vice president for clinical operations, the chief nursing officer, the quality improvement staff, the infection prevention team, the intensive care unit directors, pharmacy staff, supply chain management, and the information technology department. He estimated that this involvement cost a total of $1 million (provided in kind by HCA), which was in addition to the $2 million provided by the study's federal sponsor.

EHRs Are Necessary, But Not Sufficient

Platt noted that although EHRs hold much promise, in practice, EHRs can be difficult to use for research. One reason for this is that they are usually different in each health care system, even if they are obtained from the same commercial vendor. One way around this lack of interoperability is to extract information from the EHR system on a regular basis. This information can then be transformed and analyzed separately and in a secure setting behind the organization's firewall, which addresses Health Insurance Portability and Accountability Act and other privacy concerns. However, he noted that although data can be removed from EHRs, the placement of information back into EHRs, which would be needed to run a clinical trial, can be even more difficult.

Platt commented that the information from EHRs is often insufficient for use in clinical studies because EHRs cannot provide information about the care received by participants outside of the organization. He suggested that administrative data from health care insurers are an often undervalued source of information, especially if they can be linked to EHR data. Administrative data provide information about the care delivered across the entire spectrum of health care locations, are available for large populations, and are more standardized than most EHR data.

Organizational Consortia Are Often Required to Conduct LSTs

Many of the important topics that LSTs could address will require consortia of organizations to make reasonable progress, but the formation of consortia raises issues concerning governance and data sharing. Consortia are also expensive to build and maintain, Platt said. He discussed the benefits of distributed information networks, in which aggregate information, rather than individual patient data, can be shared and queries can be run behind organizational firewalls. In these systems, such as the Mini-Sentinel system of the U.S. Food and Drug Administration (FDA), the cancer Biomedical Informatics Grid (caBIG) system of the National Institutes of Health, the Scalable Partnering Network for Clinical Effectiveness Research of the Agency for Healthcare Research and Quality, and the Health Maintenance Organization Research Network, researchers can submit a question through a secure portal and receive the answer without having to access protected health information about individuals.

POINT-OF-CARE TRIALS USING EHR PLATFORMS

Ryan E. Ferguson presented an example of an LST that VA is carrying out using its EHR system. He described the problems that VA faced with the inefficiency of evidence creation and the failure of the research enterprise to meet the information needs of the health care system.

VA's solution was to create a learning health care system in which important clinical questions were identified and the answers could be determined through studies using VA's EHR system: the Veterans Health

Information Systems and Technology Architecture (VistA). The concept for the program is that in situations in which clinical equipoise exists between drug or intervention choices, a substantial portion of the operations of a trial to assess the question being asked could be conducted by the clinical staff as part of providing regular health care to VA beneficiaries. These LSTs could be implemented entirely within VistA, including participant identification and enrollment, consent and randomization, and data capture and management. The results learned from the trial would then become part of the decision support included in VistA.

Ferguson detailed how VA investigated the feasibility of an EHR-based point-of-care approach by conducting a pilot study comparing the use of sliding-scale versus weight-based protocols for insulin administration in diabetic patients. The study's primary endpoint was length of stay, and the secondary endpoints were rates of inpatient glycemic control and readmission within 30 days. Ferguson reported that the pilot study demonstrated the feasibility of conducting point-of-care trials by use of the EHR by finding high rates of acceptance by the providers and patients participating in the study and rates of participation higher than those usually seen in RCTs.

Ferguson closed his presentation by reflecting on VA experiences to draw broader implications for LSTs. He highlighted that it is important that the questions being asked be driven by the information needs of clinical practice and pointed out that this approach is particularly well suited to answer certain questions. He characterized these questions as ones that are asked when options between approved products and interventions with well-described toxicity are being considered, questions whose answers can be provided by measurement of objectively identifiable endpoints, and questions that can be answered with a minimal need for study-specific visits.

Looking ahead to the requirements and priorities for the generation of more evidence at the point of care, he noted that it will be important to rethink the relationship between research and clinical care, that buy-in from providers and the leaders of health care systems is key, and that a rational approach to regulatory oversight will be crucial.

OBTAINING RESEARCH-QUALITY DATA FROM EHRs

Rebecca Daniels Kush began her presentation by highlighting one of the major challenges to the efficiency of current clinical trials: the continued use of paper records and the multiple varied systems used across clinical sites. She described a number of resources currently available to streamline research studies, highlighting the fact that although these resources have the potential to be disruptive, most have not been widely implemented.

She focused her comments on the concept of eSource, which allows the collection of clinical research information entirely by electronic means without the use of paper forms while meeting existing clinical research regulations. The use of eSource, she noted, would make it easier for clinicians to conduct clinical research and would enable the extensive use of data that are collected only once.

Kush described the process used by the eSource Data Interchange (eSDI) Initiative in partnership with FDA. A multidisciplinary working group identified 12 requirements that would allow the use of eSource while still following all international regulatory rules.

The next step, Kush detailed, was part of the FDA's Critical Path Initiative, specifically, development of a minimal core data set with data in 18 categories (domains) common to all research protocols. This standard was published in 2008 and is called Clinical Data Acquisition Standards Harmonization (CDASH). An interoperability specification (specifying three standards: the continuity of care document, the retrieve form for data capture [RFD], and CDASH) was then developed through the Office of the National Coordinator for Health Information Technology of the U.S. Department of Health and Human Services as a means to obtain a common set of core research data elements to be readily exchanged between EHRs and clinical research systems. This specification was published in 2010.

Another important development was the establishment of a transport standard, called ODM, which contains audit trail information in the metadata (to support regulations described in the *Code of Federal Regulations* [21 CFR 11]). This audit trail information includes who entered the data and, if they were changed, what data were changed and who changed them, why, and when. ODM is an XML standard that carries CDASH content along with the audit trail information. The RFD standard integration profile streamlines the work flow for the population of electronic case report forms from EHRs.

As an example she highlighted the streamlining of reporting of adverse drug events (ADEs) from EHRs evaluated in the ADE Spontaneous Triggered Event Reporting project conducted by Pfizer and Harvard. That study used RFD to facilitate adverse event reporting and found that the time that it takes to make such a report was greatly decreased (from ~34 minutes to less than 1 minute), thus resulting in the reporting of many more adverse events by clinicians.

Kush explained that RFD, ODM, and CDASH do not depend on the particular EHR being used and that all of these pieces are available to support the establishment of a paperless eSource system for adverse event reporting and research.

In 2012, FDA issued guidance to the industry on data from electronic sources for clinical research, or eSource, citing that such guidance would help ensure the reliability, quality, integrity, and traceability of data from electronic sources. Kush noted that despite the maturity of the resources that she described, guidance from FDA, support from EHR vendors, and demonstrations done at industry meetings, a clinical research study of eSource has still not been done with EHRs.

She concluded her presentation with a call for sponsors to step up and take advantage of these disruptive advances that have been shown to increase research efficiency and data quality.

BUILDING REUSABLE RESEARCH NETWORKS

Carole M. Lannon's presentation covered reusable research networks, which are collaborative research and quality improvement arrangements among health care organizations that can be used for multiple purposes by different stakeholders. These networks are evolving toward the learning health care system model. Her organization, the Cincinnati Children's Hospital Medical Center, is involved in five national networks: one focused on patient safety, one focused on perinatal health, and three focused on disease.

Lannon explained that the concept behind these networks is that clinicians and researchers can learn from a much larger base of patients than they would encounter in their home institution alone. They can examine the outcomes of widely varying diagnostic and treatment practices and identify factors that lead to better outcomes. They can conduct clinical trials with much larger populations, which is especially important for pediatric care and research on diseases in the pediatric population, because the incidence of disease in pediatric populations is relatively low. Network members can undertake quality improvement efforts on the basis of research and real-time feedback as well as maintain certification credit for their participation.

Lannon presented results from ImproveCareNow, the network that has been in existence the longest that focuses on improving care for inflammatory bowel disease (IBD) for children and adolescents. She showed how, over a 4-year period, the rate of remission for IBD among some 50 children's hospitals has increased from less than 50 percent to nearly 80 percent. In another network, the 20 largest maternity hospitals in Ohio were able to reduce the rate of scheduled deliveries at between 36 and 38 completed weeks without a medical indication, shifting more than 25,000 births from preterm to term over 4 years and saving an estimated 500 neonatal intensive care unit admissions and between $15 million and $20 million. Eight Ohio children's hospitals were able to reduce the rate of surgical site infections from 4.4 to 1.7 percent, reducing the number of children harmed by about 31 a year, with a cost savings of about $680,000 a year.

Lannon presented three prerequisites for maintaining a stable learning network able to support multiple projects over time. First was a focus on outcomes. She explained that this engages patients, clinicians, and researchers and united them in their efforts to achieve something meaningful. The second focus was building a community of engaged patients, families, clinicians, and researchers through a variety of communication mechanisms and by inclusion of patients and families in governance and research. She described the learning process that they are going through to build a community, including the use of social network sites for patients to connect and share stories and for patients, families, clinicians, and researchers to collaborate effectively. The third factor is the effective use of technology, especially for more efficient data collection and use. Lannon described efforts that they are undertaking so that data entered once can be fed into automated processes to determine the proper clinical care for patients with chronic conditions, processes of measurement for quality improvement and learning, and data quality improvement processes and so that data can be used for research at population and individual levels.

Lannon discussed some of the challenges that these networks face. They include variations in institutional review boards across sites, which have led to the use of a federated institutional review board model, as well as time challenges for clinicians. Lannon also pointed to a number of trends that could improve the effectiveness of learning networks. She mentioned trends in health information technology that will enable large aggregate sets of data to be pulled from EHRs and even the use of patient sensors, as well as the exploitation of opportunities for distributed and collaborative production, in which patients and clinicians can work together to quickly tests what approaches work.

6

Ethical and Privacy Policy Issues

KEY SPEAKER THEMES

Califf

- Policy constraints are currently a greater barrier to large simple trials (LSTs) than technical limitations, which have largely been resolved.

Faden

- The current ethical framework for clinical research focuses on the risks of research and ignores the risks of clinical care practices, most of which are based on weak evidence.
- A new ethical framework is needed that allows the joining of regular clinical care and research activities, including LSTs, by appropriately balancing the risks and benefits of research when the safety and effectiveness of routine clinical practices are often unknown.

McGraw

- Current privacy regulations may unnecessarily hinder the needed reuses of clinical data for learning purposes because they more stringently regulate activities that fall under the definition of research intended to contribute to generalizable knowledge and only minimally regulate activities considered to be routine, such as treatment and internal operations.

- A new, more rational approach to the oversight of the use of patient data should depend on trade-offs between expected benefits and risks to patients and should be developed through the use of the basic principles of fair information practices.

INTRODUCTION

Large simple trials (LSTs), like all clinical trials, are governed by policies designed to protect the health, safety, and privacy of participants. The session of the workshop described in this chapter focused on whether these policies are appropriate or need to be revised in a way that still protects participants adequately but facilitates the conduct of LSTs as an important evidence-generating activity in the learning health care system.

Robert M. Califf, director of the Duke Translational Medicine Institute, professor of medicine, and vice chancellor for clinical and translational research at the Duke University Medical Center, provided an overview of the current policy context and highlighted issues that might be candidates for review and revision to better balance ethical and privacy concerns to facilitate LSTs. Ruth R. Faden, Philip Franklin Wagley Professor of Biomedical Ethics and executive director of the Johns Hopkins Berman Institute of Bioethics at The Johns Hopkins University, spoke about the shortfalls of the current ethical framework that guides oversight of clinical research and suggested that a new one might be necessary. Deven McGraw, director of the Health Privacy Project at the Center for Democracy and Technology, discussed the development and promotion of more workable privacy and security protections for electronic personal health information.

POLICY OVERVIEW

Robert M. Califf gave an overview of some of the major policy barriers to the more widespread performance of LSTs. He pointed out that the vision of a national clinical research system that extended into the community was not a new concept; in fact, it had been a 10-year goal of the National Institutes of Health (NIH) Roadmap in 2002. Although most (85 percent) recommendations in clinical practice guidelines are based on low-quality evidence, the current clinical trials enterprise cannot produce results fast enough to close the gap. Noting that technology is no longer the limiting factor in conducting LSTs and producing this evidence, he asked, what is preventing the conduct of LSTs?

Califf posited that the barriers to implementation are not technical because it is possible to collect standardized reliable data from electronic records. Rather, the barriers have to do with policy constraints. Califf suggested that a window of opportunity to revise policies that impede LSTs and other clinical research exists, because the leaders of federal health agencies have shown that they are open to reforming the national clinical trials system, health care providers have proved willing to participate if the studies answer questions important to them and they do not lose money, and the experience with potential trial participants is that the majority of individuals will participate if they are asked.

So, the question is, what policies will more quickly allow the selection of standardized, reliable data that could serve as a backbone for a learning system that, Califf would argue, includes LSTs? Califf cited his experiences as principal investigator of the NIH-funded Health Systems Research Collaboratory Coordinating Center, where he was charged with helping pilot projects navigate these challenges. He indicated that those involved in the pilot projects contend that the top issues are interfacing with the health system and regulatory ethics.

Looking at the challenges of interactions with health systems, Califf asked, what policies can motivate health systems administrators to participate in research, ensure that the trials done answer questions of interest to clinicians and patients, and, assuming that the clinical trials are relevant, motivate providers to participate? Highlighting the major regulatory changes that are needed, Califf asked if the ethical review and institutional requirements for oversight of research could be streamlined without putting research participants at undue risk and if the U.S. Food and Drug Administration could actively encourage streamlining of procedures. He suggested that key federal agencies could encourage novel approaches to reviews by institutional review board and informed consent, highlighting the issue of dealing with cluster randomization as a major issue if LSTs are to be widespread in the community.

Califf closed his presentation by asking whether, given the hurt that the current system has caused patients by its failure to answer critical questions, the underlying construct of separation of research and practice is appropriate and reasonable.

ETHICAL ISSUES IN BRINGING RESEARCH AND CARE CLOSER TOGETHER

Ruth R. Faden addressed whether the separation of clinical research and clinical care is ethically appropriate. She explained that the current framework for health care ethics was developed in the 1970s, when abuses of participants in research projects were salient. This was exemplified by the Tuskegee research experiment conducted from 1932 to 1972, in which subjects were infected with the spirochete that causes syphilis without their knowledge and treatment was withheld, even after penicillin was proven to be an effective cure. In the context of the Tuskegee study, regulations to protect human subjects in health research, principally, the Common Rule, were developed, and the Office for Human Research Protections was established in the U.S. Department of Health Services.

Given this context, the framework for regulation of clinical research with human participants was based on a sharp distinction between research and clinical care, since the focus was protecting individuals' rights and interests when they participated in clinical research.

Faden noted that the concept of a learning health system calls this division into question, as it proposes that it is essential to learn from care, therefore integrating research and practice. Reconciliation of the division requires a different way of thinking about the relationship between research ethics and clinical ethics. One of the bases for this distinction is the assumption that research places patients at higher risk than regular clinical care. However, she noted that many approaches, such as LSTs, are likely to challenge this assumption. It is now known that many commonly accepted clinical practices have a weak evidence base, and some have been proven to have no benefit or even to be harmful to patients. To reduce the harm done to patients, the current framework, Faden argued, constrains the ability to conduct research that could potentially demonstrate that some commonly used treatments are less effective than other treatments or even harmful compared with other treatments.

Faden noted that the moral requirement to show respect for patients and honor their necessary role in this research also exists. This, she explained, has implications for how consent is thought about in a learning health system, as alternative approaches to individual consent must also fulfill this requirement.

Faden and other health ethicists have been working for several years to develop new ethical guidelines that would support a learning health care system. She noted that these guidelines would have to include a sense of reciprocity in which researchers commit to respect for patients and patients commit to contribute to the process of knowledge generation. She suggested that this reciprocity must be expressed through practices, such as transparency, disclosure, and oversight, that are acceptable to patients and involve patients in a different way than is currently the norm, but these practices remain to be determined.

CHALLENGES WITH THE CLINICAL TRIAL PROCESS

Deven McGraw's presentation about privacy issues paralleled Faden's, in that McGraw found that the distinction between research and clinical practice in current regulations stands in the way of the conduct of LSTs and other important clinical research as part of the process of providing regular health care. She described how the Health Insurance Portability and Accountability Act distinguishes the use of patient data as either routine and nonroutine. Patient data can be routinely used without additional authorization, for example, as a basis for patient treatment, as a basis for the treatment of another patient, or for health care operations (such as billing and quality improvement). In fact, McGraw points out, patients are not able to opt out of the use of their information for these purposes. Research, however, is considered to be a nonroutine use of data, and in most cases, researchers are required to obtain specific authorization.

The distinction between routine use and research is based on the definition of "research" as something that contributes to generalizable knowledge. This creates a situation in which, for example, the use of patient information for quality improvement is considered routine if it is kept within the treating organization but as nonroutine if the results obtained with those data are shared more broadly. McGraw pointed out that these two scenarios involve the exact same use of data in terms of what data are accessed, who accesses the data, and the questions being posed. This, she argued, is problematic for a learning health system, for which dissemination of learning is critical.

McGraw suggested two possible remedies. One, which she noted would be problematic, would be to make a case to consider routine individual data uses that are currently considered nonroutine. An alternative approach would be to develop criteria to guide the use of data so that oversight is decided according to the trade-offs between the benefits to patients expected from the use of those data and the risks that the data might be leaked and misused. In this setting, issues of how many and which people would have access to the data, how individually identifiable the data are, and what mechanisms for data security will be used would drive oversight, rather than whether the results will be shared. McGraw suggested that fair information practices, which are already the basis for most uses of personal data, could serve as a good foundation for the legal frameworks and systems of accountability necessary to put this into practice. For example, oversight would emphasize that the data be kept in the least identifiable form possible and that the fewest possible number of people possible have access to the data. Mechanisms such as distributed networks could help ensure that the data are used effectively without a loss control over their use.

McGraw noted that as different approaches are considered, piloting of their use and the study of their effects will be crucial to the development of practical approaches and to appeal to policy makers as well as patient and consumer groups to permit the use of patient data. Similar to the ethics guiding research with human subjects in a learning health care system, new ways of engaging patients that respect their right to have a say in what research is done and to learn how their data will be used to improve health care would be needed.

7

Research Partner Perspectives

KEY SPEAKER THEMES

Roach

- Changing the way patients are thought about, as consumers of research rather than just as study subjects, is a core principle for engaging patients in research.
- Better information and decision support are needed to help patients make informed decisions about their participation in research.
- Sharing of trial results and reconnection with trial participants show respect for participants and acknowledge their efforts, creating satisfied customers who will describe the opportunity to participate in research to others.

Go

- The current context of health care delivery, which is increasingly efficient and has higher throughput, creates both challenges and opportunities for large simple trials (LSTs).
- Electronic health records are both part of the solution and part of the problem to increasing the amount of research conducted in health care settings.

- Health care systems and health care providers have many reasons to participate more actively in research, including illuminating the many remaining unknowns in medicine and the potential competitive advantages of a learning culture.

Sandy

- LSTs can be very informative to payers because they can help answer questions about the effectiveness of treatments under real-world conditions.
- A greater speed at which questions are answered must be accompanied by a greater speed at which the findings of research are used to achieve a learning health system that promotes high-value innovation.

INTRODUCTION

For large simple trials (LSTs) to be a successful approach to generating evidence, their value must be appreciated by health care delivery systems, clinicians, patients, and payers. Health systems must weigh their participation in LSTs against the many other efforts competing for resources; clinicians, as the primary data collectors, must make time for LSTs in their already busy care schedules; patients must see LSTs to be worthy of the collection of information about them; and payers must see LSTs to be the producers of useful knowledge. This chapter summarizes presentations from these perspectives.

Nancy Roach, chair of the board of directors of Fight Colorectal Cancer gave the patient perspective. She founded Fight Colorectal Cancer in 2005 after her mother-in-law was diagnosed with colorectal cancer. Alan S. Go, chief of cardiovascular and metabolic conditions, Kaiser Permanente Division of Research, and Northern California regional medical director for clinical trials at The Permanente Medical Group, offered the perspectives of both health care professionals and the health care delivery system. The perspective of the payer community was provided by Lewis G. Sandy, senior vice president for clinical advancement at UnitedHealth Group.

PATIENT PERSPECTIVE

Nancy Roach began her presentation by highlighting the disconnect between the assumptions that most people make about the research system and the reality. Noting that most people are not exposed to the research system until they are at an extremely vulnerable moment, when they are sick, she asked how the equation can be changed so that people care about research and are willing to listen when they are called upon to participate.

She said that people believe in health care research and are willing to participate in clinical trials if they are approached as partners in research and consumers of the findings of research rather than as research subjects. An important part of the signaling of this difference is language, for example, through the use of the word "participant" instead of the word "subject." She suggested that changing the way in which patients are thought about, as consumers of research rather than just study subjects, should change the way in which research is developed by placement of the priority on what is important to patients.

Roach highlighted the need for better information and decision support for patients, so that patients can make informed decisions about their participation in research. She also emphasized the importance of reconnecting with trial participants, to show them respect and acknowledge their efforts. These, she said, are all approaches to creating satisfied customers and research partners who will spread the word about their involvement and bring the opportunity to participate in research to the attention of others.

HEALTH SYSTEMS/CLINICIAN PERSPECTIVE

Alan S. Go began his presentation by putting the issue of LSTs into the context that health care delivery systems currently face: the need for greater efficiency and higher throughput. Changes in the health care system are increasing competition, squeezing revenues, and making health care delivery systems more efficient. These changes make streamlined evidence generation activities such as LSTs more desirable but also potentially less feasible. He also noted that the goals of the major stakeholders—the health care delivery system, clinicians, researchers, sponsors, and patients—are often different. Go noted that health systems must balance a number of competing priorities. The goals include the provision of care of optimal quality, improved patient access, increased provider efficiency, better electronic health record (EHR) systems, and maintenance of revenues and strategic investments.

Go noted that EHRs have been both a solution and part of the problem and that they are not a panacea for clinical research but are certainly a promising part of the solution. First, EHR systems are different; even an EHR system provided by the same company is adapted to some extent to each health care system that uses it. Second, health systems have many efforts vying for the use of their EHR systems, making expansion of their use for clinical trials very challenging. Third, achievement of the kind of standardized data collection suitable for clinical trials poses work flow issues and requires buy-in from health care providers. He concluded that

EHRs will be part of a solution for certain kinds of questions but not for every question and that creativity will be necessary to determine how best to use the EHR for data collection, randomization, and other reasons but that it is unlikely to be the only solution.

However, Go argued, health systems and health care providers have many reasons to participate more actively in trials. For one, many things in medicine remain unknown. LSTs could be an opportunity to show that, when done right, randomization is a very important design and that the culture of randomization or learning can be an advantage to a health care delivery system.

Go reflected on important ways forward, including the suggestion that research sponsors get early systematic input from health systems about the questions of most import to them rather than relying solely on areas of interest to researchers. He noted that incentives to clinicians and health care systems are needed to ensure participation and that health care systems should be challenged to think about forming LST consortia at regional or national levels.

In closing, Go encouraged the field to think about identifying questions that would be wins for all stakeholders—health systems, sponsors, clinicians, and patients—and suggested several examples, including diagnostic and management strategies for lower back pain.

PAYER PERSPECTIVE

Lewis G. Sandy began by explaining that payers like UnitedHealthcare are always trying to determine when a service is proven to be cost-effective and no longer experimental or investigational and thus eligible for insurance coverage. They are also always interested in supporting high-value innovation, even if it would be disruptive.

Sandy noted that questions that are common among payers concern effectiveness and safety: Does it work? How strong is the evidence? Is it safe? What specific populations would benefit and which would not? Does the proposed procedure, service, or drug improve health outcomes? What are all the advantages, possible harms, and alternatives? LSTs can help answer these questions under real-world conditions, but such questions cannot be answered under the highly specific conditions of a traditional randomized controlled trial. LSTs may also provide answers more rapidly, if it is assumed that reliable randomization exists and that the cohorts are truly comparable, that is, if not too many patients decide not to participate.

He said that it is important to address these questions not only for payers but also for all the stakeholders, including patients, clinicians, and health care delivery systems. He urged all parties to work together to promote LSTs and other approaches to high-value innovation.

Sandy pointed out that some important questions can be answered by the use of approaches other than LSTs, for example, by a prospective or a retrospective observational study. Also, he said, not only do answers about interventions need to be obtained more rapidly, but also the use of proven interventions, such as colorectal screening, which is reaching only 60 percent of the target population, needs to be increased. This is the goal of a learning health system. Clinical registries can be useful here, he said. They not only provide a good infrastructure for collecting and analyzing data but also provide a potentially effective dissemination mechanism to rapidly incorporate learning into clinical practice guidelines and build best practices into clinical decision support systems.

8

The Randomized Evaluations of Accepted Choices in Treatment Trials[1]

KEY SPEAKER THEMES

van Staa

- Despite the advantages of a single health care system and electronic health records, the Randomized Evaluations of Accepted Choices in Treatment trials face many of the same challenges that large simple trials (LSTs) conducted in the United States encounter.
- Ways to encourage more LSTs need to be found because of the huge costs of not testing alternative treatments that are commonly prescribed.
- To get to simpler trials, governance that protects participants as well as facilitates important research is required.

INTRODUCTION

The keynote address was delivered during lunch on the second day of the workshop by Tjeerd-Pieter van Staa. van Staa is the head of research for Clinical Practice Research Datalink (CPRD), which is an observational data

[1] The views expressed during the keynote address are those of Tjeerd-Pieter van Staa and do not reflect the official policy or position of the Medicines and Healthcare Products Regulatory Agency.

and interventional research service jointly funded by the United Kingdom's National Institute for Health Research and the Medicines and Healthcare Products Regulatory Agency.

RANDOMIZED EVALUATIONS OF ACCEPTED CHOICES IN TREATMENT TRIALS

Randomized Evaluations of Accepted Choices in Treatment (REACT) is the title of an effort launched by CPRD to conduct pragmatic, large simple trials (van Staa, 2011). The goal of REACT is to test alternative clinical interventions commonly prescribed by physicians that have not been evaluated for their comparative effectiveness through the use of data routinely collected in the single electronic health record (EHR) system used by the United Kingdom's National Health Service. van Staa began by noting that the motivation for the program lay with the National Health Service's finding that participants in randomized controlled trials (RCTs) are not necessarily representative of the general population and that the actions of patients and clinicians in RCTs are not necessarily those of patients and clinicians in everyday clinical practice. In other words, RCTs can lack external validity. van Staa illustrated this be mentioning as examples the drugs Celebrex and Vioxx, which were approved on the basis of high-quality RCTs. However, when they were routinely prescribed to members of the general population—most of whom would not have qualified to participate in the RCTs, he noted—serious side effects emerged. Another problem that van Staa identified is the lack of evidence for many common treatments for prevalent diseases. If a given condition has more than one commonly prescribed treatment, physicians and patients do not have a basis for knowing which one is safer or more effective.

One of the missions of CPRD is to use data that are routinely collected in the EHR during care to conduct RCTs of common treatments while imposing a minimum burden on clinicians or patients. CPRD can do this because it has arrangements with a large number of general clinical practices to report health care data regularly. Currently, CPRD has records on about 5 million patients, about 8 percent of the patient population served by the National Health Service, and this database is updated monthly. van Staa noted that CPRD uses pseudoanonymized data and can link its data sets to other data sets, such as hospital data, disease registries, and death certificates.

At this time, CPRD is conducting two small REACT trials to test the feasibility of this approach. One study, RETRO-PRO, involving about 300 patients, is comparing two popular statins, simvastatin and atorvastatin, which have each been previously tested in RCTs against placebo. e-LUNG, the other study, involving 150 patients, looks at antibiotic use in patients with chronic obstructive pulmonary disease (COPD). Some clinicians pre-scribe antibiotics for patients who experience a COPD exacerbation, and others do not. However, little evidence on the clinical effect of antibiotics on COPD exacerbations currently exists.

van Staa described the trial processes in more detail. He noted that participants in eLUNG must be recruited in real time, when they are hav-ing an exacerbation, which is done through the use of flagging software in the EHR that alerts the clinician that the patient may be eligible for the trial. In contrast, for RETRO-PRO, participating clinicians are sent a list of potentially eligible participants derived from information in the EHR database. Despite the very inclusive nature of the trials, van Staa noted that the trials had few eligibility criteria that had to be evaluated. In RETRO-PRO, they included whether the patients had used a statin before and whether they were at high risk for cardiovascular disease. If neither of these applied, patients were randomized into the trial. In the case of both trials, he explained, participating patients must consent to be included in the study. After this point, clinicians and patients are generally followed unobtrusively. Follow-up information is generally collected from the rou-tinely reported EHR data, unless some anomaly or other question arises, in which case CPRD researchers can contact the clinician for information.

Although REACT trials have the advantage of working in a single very large health care system with a single EHR, in which uniform patient in-formation is continuously reported to a central data bank, they have faced challenges, which van Staa enumerated. One major obstacle is the burden-some requirements for informed consent and regulatory reporting oversight imposed by research governance. van Staa detailed how CPRD proposed a one-page informed consent form, which the ethics committee would not approve and insisted on lengthening. Additionally, regulators required re-ports every 7 or 15 days, depending on the item. The researchers argued that reports every 7 or 15 days would be burdensome on the clinicians and that monthly reports would be adequate, given the low degree of risk of the interventions. Clinicians were also required to undergo training in the protocol, despite CPRD's argument that training in prescribing statins was probably not necessary and would be an additional burden on clinicians.

van Staa noted that another problem that the REACT trials face is the lack of incentives for clinicians to participate, given their already very busy care schedules. Possibly as a result of this, CPRD found that relatively few potentially eligible patients were being recruited. A few weeks earlier, for example, van Staa reported that 10 patients had been recruited in a certain practice but that another 260 who could have been recruited were not.

Variable recording and coding of health care data, especially across the linked data sets, is another challenge to the REACT trials, as are variations in practice across National Health Service sites. For example, one of the issues that RETRO-PRO faced was a price difference between simvastatin and atorvastatin. Many local NHS organizations require clinicians to use the cheaper one, simvastatin, and will not make an exception for research, even though the research might have implications for cost-effectiveness. Because of this, van Staa shared, in some locations, clinicians prescribe atorvastatin for the 3 months of the study and then switch the patient back to simvastatin, preventing long-term follow-up.

Despite the many challenges that the REACT trials have faced, van Staa concluded with the observation that ways must be found to make LSTs work because not doing them has a cost to patients. For example, a patient who currently has a COPD exacerbation receives an antibiotic or does not receive an antibiotic, depending on which clinician he or she happens to see. Instead, he said, clinicians should know whether antibiotics work or not. Regarding the sharp ethical distinction between research and clinical practice discussed earlier in the workshop, van Staa posited that research on chronic conditions, such as COPD, would provide a benefit to the individual participant as well as a generalizable benefit, because the participant would continue to have the condition after the trial ends.

REFERENCE

van Staa, T., B. Goldacre, M. Gulliford, J. Cassell, M. Pirmohamed, A. Taweel, B. Delaney, and L. Smeeth. 2011. Randomised Evaluations of Accepted Choices in Treatment (REACT) trials: Large-scale pragmatic trials within databases of routinely collected electronic healthcare records, abstr. A104. Presented at the 12th Clinical Trials Methodology Conference.

9

Strategies Going Forward

During the final session of the workshop, individual participants reflected on the workshop presentations and discussions and discussed actions that they believed were important to achieving progress in the areas discussed. The suggestions made by individual participants covered five broad thematic areas: learning-ready records, the availability of a network for the development of questions, science stewardship, facilitative oversight, and the presence of a learning culture.

LEARNING-READY RECORDS

Throughout the workshop, many speakers and participants who spoke commented on the key role of electronic health records (EHRs) in large simple trials (LSTs). Their use was often cited to be critical to carrying out large trials that are integrated into the care setting. However, Richard Platt, in particular, cautioned against the notion that they are a panacea, noting that in their current state they can be quite difficult to use.

This discussion pointed to more interoperable, learning-ready records as a priority for progress. Approaches to achieving learning-ready records included enabling all records to collect a minimum data set designed to support maximum improvements in health care and the more widespread use and piloting of minimal data resources already in existence. The identification of such a data set was suggested to be an important first step in this endeavor, which would require the engagement of multiple stakeholders as well as national leadership to consider issues such as balancing the burden of data collection with clinical burdens and work flows.

Some progress toward the electronic collection of minimal data sets is already under way, as Rebecca Daniels Kush of Clinical Data Interchange Standards Consortium (CDISC) detailed. CDISC's work to facilitate the collection of data for clinical trials from EHRs was cited as critical progress toward making the maximum use of digital health data for research.

In addition to the collection of the appropriate information to support learning, it was highlighted by several workshop participants that spoke that effective data sharing will be crucial to obtaining the amount of data needed for LSTs. Data sharing of this magnitude will require technical as well as policy solutions.

Several participants pointed to the interoperability of data to be a critical component to ensure that data are comparable across sites. Approaches to the sharing of data, such as distributed networks, that do not require the data to leave the originating institution were highlighted to be particularly promising. These challenges that the participants who spoke identified, however, are far from resolved and will require sustained innovation and continued capacity development.

Some participants, particularly Tim Ferris, pointed to the move toward accountable care organizations, which require the collection, sharing, and use of more data, as well as a focus on outcomes, as potential levers for progress toward the achievement of more learning-ready records. Still, collaborative, national, and global efforts to continue progress on the challenges of interoperability, data sharing, and standardization were priorities that participants who spoke mentioned often.

NETWORK FOR QUESTION DEVELOPMENT

Throughout the workshop, several participants and speakers pointed to the importance of the use of appropriate methodological approaches to answer research questions. Much discussion was had about the sorts of questions that LSTs are best suited to answer, with the understanding that all approaches have advantages and disadvantages. Stating that much of the research currently being conducted does not produce the evidence needed to inform decision making and that many basic effectiveness questions are left unanswered, several participants noted the opportunity to strengthen the evidence base in a way that can inform population-level questions and, ultimately, individual care decisions through the broader use of LSTs. Participants noted that the development of a national capacity to conduct LSTs could be accompanied by an ongoing capacity to elicit, refine, and triage questions to be addressed.

Several factors influencing the prioritization of research questions were discussed. These included functions of the nature of the question, such as the expected size of the effect and outcomes, in addition to issues of stakeholder engagement.

References were made to the recent efforts made by the Patient-Centered Outcomes Research Institute (PCORI) to elicit research topics from a wide range of stakeholders and how such efforts could be a potential model to obtain questions to be answered by LSTs. Joe V. Selby, from PCORI, noted that no single legitimate source for research questions exists. He highlighted that although patients are beginning to be engaged in these efforts, clinicians and health care systems, crucial stakeholders in this work, are currently the least prepared to participate.

Among the issues raised were the different and often contrasting interests held by different stakeholders, as was echoed for the health care system level during Alan S. Go's presentation during the workshop, and the need to balance these interests against the importance of maintaining scientific rigor. Several participants highlighted the need for inclusive governance structures and policies to support dialogues about prioritization.

SCIENCE STEWARDSHIP

The continued development and innovation of methods for the conduct of LSTs were key issues of discussion among several workshop participants and speakers. Efforts to affix a single, rigid definition to LSTs were discouraged, reflecting both the evolving landscape and the acknowledgment that one size does not fit all. Robert Temple suggested that rather than focus on one research approach, a theme of the workshop was the need for simpler trials overall and that one potential use for LSTs is the follow-up of hypotheses generated from observational studies.

As the infrastructural and policy capacity to conduct LSTs develops, several participants highlighted that methodological innovation must keep pace but that scientific rigor must be maintained. A theme of Rachel E. Sherman's presentation, that the focus should be on producing good-quality data that answers the question being asked rather than on the selection of a particular methodology for the sake of it, was echoed by other workshop participants. One of the challenges to this, highlighted by Ralph I. Horwitz, is the need to get a better sense of what needs to be done to get to credible evidence in the variety of diverse situations in which evidence from LSTs will be used.

Several of the challenges to the broader use of LSTs that workshop participants who spoke highlighted dealt with current reward structures within the research community. A number of speakers and individual discussants pointed to the need for incentives for value rather than incentives for volume of studies (in which volume covers both the number of studies and the amount of data collected), which are major contributors to the unnecessary complexity of clinical studies. The current approaches, they said, have resulted in the conduct of many low-quality studies without sufficient thought being given to study efficiency, including the placement of limits on the amount of data collected, the value of the questions asked to key stakeholders, or the utility of the results.

Many participants discussed the need to develop metrics, potentially for use by research funders, to assess the progress of research efforts toward these goals and reward those that make effective use of resources and contribute meaningfully to a useful evidence base for care and decision making.

FACILITATIVE OVERSIGHT

Much of the discussion around policy challenges to the broader use of LSTs in the United States centered on the need for clear and facilitative oversight. Several presentations touched on the underlying reasons for the current complexity and inefficiencies of the clinical research enterprise. These included discussions over the shift of the focus of clinical trials from acute to chronic diseases and the collection of more genetic data but also highlighted the lack of understanding between researchers and regulatory and oversight organizations.

In the case of research on regulated products, speakers and individual participants spoke of a sense that many of the data were collected in response to a perception that they could be required by regulatory agencies, such as the U.S. Food and Drug Administration (FDA), and that the unnecessary collection of such large amounts of data greatly increased the cost and complexity of clinical trials. This perception was countered by comments from FDA officials that such fears are largely unfounded. Many individual participants highlighted that for the streamlined approaches required by LSTs to be more widely used in the assessment of regulated products, this communication and understanding gap must be closed. Clear, specific guidance from FDA on the use of LSTs and streamlining of clinical trials were highlighted as important first steps in this effort. Other strategies discussed included better training of study case managers to break cycles of unnecessary or defensive data collection.

Discussions of the need for clear, facilitative oversight also extended to the bodies responsible for research protections, including sharing of data. Ruth R. Faden's presentation highlighted the reasons that the current framework for ethical oversight is no longer suitable to meet the requirements of a learning health system, particularly as it deals with learning from the delivery of health care. She suggested that a new ethics framework that supports learning and protects patients will be necessary to show respect for patients and honor their role in research.

A number of individual participants highlighted the crucial need for a research governance regime that meets these goals of protecting patients while allowing the kind of learning from care that LSTs can facilitate.

Informed consent was one specific area for potential improvement that several participants highlighted. Suggestions on ways to improve informed consent included improving and shortening consent forms, rethinking the requirement for informed consent in situations limited to the use of patient information, and leveraging electronic platform to obtain portable legal consent.

Discussions of data sharing and privacy oversight policies followed similar themes. Deven McGraw's presentation and comments from several participants highlighted the misplaced focus on differentiation of operations and research as a way to guide oversight of data sharing. Alternative suggestions of ways to protect patient information while facilitating learning processes included the application of fair information principles and keeping in mind patient expectations about what their data will be used for.

LEARNING CULTURE

A theme of the discussion on what it will take to achieve the greater use of LSTs that arose often throughout the workshop was the need to move toward a culture of continuous learning in which every clinical care encounter is an opportunity for learning. Comments and reflections on discussions about the technical challenges facing LSTs often concluded that although work remains to be done in these areas, the real barriers are those of culture, including resistance to the use of randomization.

Individual workshop participants highlighted the need for leadership from the top that reflects the principles of learning from the provision of clinical care, the need to embed this concept into the organizational mission, and the need to use efficient, integrated methods to develop evidence that is useful for decision making. Approaches to achieving the goals that were discussed included training of support staff and clinicians, alignment of incentives, and the creation of incentives when necessary to ensure that everyone, including clinicians and patients, has a business case for participation in research.

Some participants called for efforts to fully engage clinicians and patients at all levels of the learning process: question identification, study design, implementation, and dissemination. Specifically, the need to address aversions to participating in integrated trials by clinicians who might perceive these to be risky propositions was mentioned. The call for patient engagement included the need to reframe patients as consumers of research rather than research subjects, the need for transparent dialogues about the risks and benefits of participation in research, and the complementary ethical responsibilities of clinicians and systems to protect patients and of patients to participate in the kinds of learning activities that will ultimately benefit them and others like them. The need to develop careful and respectful communication strategies was highlighted to be an important component of these engagement efforts.

Finally, several individual participants highlighted the need to educate the end users of the evidence produced by approaches like LSTs in an effort to build awareness of the advantages of research and maximize the impact and utility of the results.

Appendix A

Workshop Agenda

**LARGE SIMPLE TRIALS AND KNOWLEDGE
GENERATION IN A LEARNING HEALTH SYSTEM**

An Institute of Medicine Workshop

November 26–27, 2012

Room 100
Keck Center
500 Fifth Street NW, Washington, DC

Roundtable on Value & Science-Driven Health Care
Forum on Drug Discovery, Development, and Translation

Meeting Objectives

1. Explore accelerating the use of large simple trials (LSTs) to improve the speed and practicality of knowledge generation for medical decision making and medical product development;
2. Consider the concepts of LST design, examples of successful LSTs, the relative advantages of LSTs, and the infrastructure needed to build LST capacity as a routine function of care;
3. Identify structural, cultural, and regulatory barriers hindering the development of an enhanced LST capacity and discuss needs and strategies in building public demand for, and participation in, LSTs; and
4. Suggest near-term strategies for accelerating progress in the uptake of LSTs in the United States.

Monday, November 26

1:00 pm   **Welcome, Introductions, and Overview**
Welcome, framing of the meeting, and agenda overview
- o Michael McGinnis (Institute of Medicine)
- o David L. DeMets (Planning Committee Co-Chair, University of Wisconsin School of Public Health)
- o Richard E. Kuntz (Planning Committee Co-Chair, Medtronic)

1:15 pm   **Introduction to Large Simple Trials**
Session chair: David L. DeMets (Planning Committee Co-Chair, University of Wisconsin School of Public Health)

➢ **Session Objectives:**
- o Set the vision for large simple trials (LSTs) as part of a learning health care system.
- o Discuss the advantages of LSTs over current trial approaches.
- o Discuss opportunities for LSTs as way to embed trials in growing digital infrastructure.

➢ **Presentations:**
- o **A vision for LSTs in the learning health system**
  Michael S. Lauer (National Heart, Lung, and Blood Institute)
- o **Opportunities and challenges for LSTs**
  Ralph I. Horwitz (GlaxoSmithKline)

➢ **Session Questions:**
1. What is an LST?
2. How would these trials fit into the larger clinical research ecosystem in a learning health care system?
3. What need would this approach to clinical trials fill? (randomized controlled trial [RCT] cost, efficiency, generalizability)
4. What are the advantages/disadvantages to this approach? (heterogeneity, subgroup analysis)
5. How does the increased adoption of electronic health records (EHRs) provide an opportunity for LSTs?
6. Are there modifications to the current design and conduct of LSTs that would enhance their value to a learning health system?

7. What are some exampleas of the areas still in need of work to realize this vision (e.g., the culture shift needed to adopt potentially disruptive technologies)?

Q&A and Open Discussion

1:55 pm **Highlighted Examples of LSTs**
Session chair: James B. Young (Cleveland Clinic)

➢ **Session Objectives:**
   o Highlight four examples of LSTs that each exemplify a different defining characteristic of LSTs.
   o Emphasize trade-offs in trial design by discussing the pros and cons, giving examples of how these play out, and suggesting alternative approaches.
   o Foreshadow the rest of the workshop by asking LST example speakers to address their experiences (successes and failures) with stakeholder engagement, infrastructure, and policy.

➢ **Presentations:**
   o Very large, population-based trial with broad inclusion criteria, high cost-efficiency, and hybrid design (mail-based plus in-clinic component)
      ▪ **VITamin D and omegA 3 triaL (VITAL)**
        JoAnn E. Manson (Harvard University)
   o Trial assessing role of waiving medication copayments for improving drug adherence and health outcomes, collaboration with health insurance company (Aetna)
      ▪ **Post-Myocardial Infarction Free Rx Event and Economic Evaluation (MI FREEE) trial**
        Niteesh K. Choudhry (Brigham and Women's Hospital)
   o Cluster randomized trial involving pediatric practices, utilization of EHR and decision support tools for obesity interventions
      ▪ **High Five for Kids Trial/Study of Technology to Accelerate Research (STAR)**
        Elsie M. Taveras (Harvard Pilgrim Health Care Institute)

       o Industry trial for regulatory approval with global component
- **Heart Outcomes Prevention Evaluation (HOPE) trial**

       P. J. Devereaux (McMaster University)

> **Session Questions:**
>
> 1. Please give a very brief introduction on the specifics of the trial and why it is considered an LST.
> 2. How does the trial address the issues of the generalizability of the evidence produced, simplification of research processes, and cost-effectiveness?
> 3. In retrospect, what were the risks and trade-offs associated with the choice of an LST design (e.g., the risk of not collecting data that could be subsequently requested)? Please discuss the pros and cons, giving examples of how these play out and suggesting alternative approaches and any design changes that you would make on the basis of the lessons learned.
> 4. What were your team's experiences (successes and failures) with the following issues, which will be discussed in further detail during the course of the workshop:
>   a. Stakeholder (health system leader, clinician, patient) engagement
>   b. Infrastructure (research infrastructure, health information technology)
>   c. Policy (privacy, consent, institutional review board issues, regulatory issues)

       Q&A and Open Discussion

3:15 pm   **Break**

3:30 pm   **Partners Perspectives on LST Uptake**
               Session chair: Joe V. Selby (Patient-Centered Outcomes Research Institute)

> **Session Objectives:**
>
> o Identify stakeholders relevant to the increased use of LSTs, focusing on patients, clinicians/health care systems, and payers, and the incentives that they face that could impede or advance uptake.

    o Engage in the issues of the most importance to stakeholders and deliberate on what it will take from each of their respective points of view.

> **Presentations:**
> > o **Patient perspective**
> > Nancy Roach (Fight Colorectal Cancer)
> > o **Health systems/clinician perspective**
> > Alan S. Go (Kaiser Permanente)
> > o **Payer perspective**
> > Lewis G. Sandy (UnitedHealth Group)

> **Session Questions:**
> 1. What are the top three issues for patients/clinicians/ payers in considering the use of an LST approach to generate clinical evidence?
> 2. What are the top three considerations for patients and clinicians in contemplating the greater integration of trials into routine care settings?
> 3. What are the top three priorities for raising the awareness and participation of patients and clinicians in trials integrated into routine care?
> 4. What are your priorities regarding the types of evidence that can be generated through LSTs?
> 5. What are the roles for health systems and payers in (a) setting priorities, (b) dedicating staff support, and (c) providing funding for LSTs in routine care settings?

    Q&A and Open Discussion

4:30 pm   **Summary and Preview of Next Day**

5:00 pm   **Adjourn**

    Tuesday, November 27

8:00 am   Coffee and light breakfast available

8:30 am   **Welcome, Brief Agenda Overview**
    Welcome, framing of the meeting, and agenda overview
      o David L. DeMets (Planning Committee Co-Chair, University of Wisconsin School of Public Health)
      o Richard E. Kuntz (Planning Committee Co-Chair, Medtronic)

8:45 am   **Infrastructure Needs**
                 Session chair: John J. Orloff (Novartis)

> ➤ **Session Objectives:**
>   - o Highlight infrastructure needs and barriers to the greater performance of LSTs.
>   - o Discuss the needs and potential approaches to merge the goals of the health care system with research, focusing on the current state and future potential of the use of EHRs as platform for LSTs.
>   - o Discuss establishment and sustainability of trial networks as an infrastructure to host and facilitate LSTs.

> ➤ **Presentations:**
>   - o **Aligning care and research to reduce burdens and improve integration**
>   Richard Platt (Harvard Pilgrim Health Care Institute)
>   - o **Point-of-care trials using EHR platforms**
>   Ryan E. Ferguson (VA Boston Healthcare System)
>   - o **Getting to comparable, computable data**
>   Rebecca Daniels Kush (Clinical Data Interchange Standards Consortium)
>   - o **Building reusable research networks**
>   Carole M. Lannon (Cincinnati Children's Hospital Center)

> ➤ **Session Questions:**
>   1. What are the current infrastructure needs for the more widespread performance of LSTs? Would you consider conducting LSTs on your network?
>   2. What opportunities and challenges in the use of EHRs as a platform for LSTs currently exist? What are the priorities for change to maximize this potential going forward? How can disruption to the delivery of health care be minimized to incentivize more practicing physicians to engage in knowledge generation?
>   3. What is the current state of the use of routinely collected clinical data for trials? What role will data standards play in the facilitation of LSTs? What are the priorities for change to maximize this potential going forward?

4. What is the current state of reusable research networks in the United States? What is their role in LSTs? What are the major opportunities and barriers to the reusable network approach? Are there alternative community-based settings with lower infrastructure costs and greater access to patients that should be considered? Are existing research networks (including perhaps CTSA institutions or PBRNs) fit for purpose? What business models (e.g., hub and spoke) would be the most effective?

Q&A and Open Discussion

10:45 am   **Break**

11:00 am   **Policy Needs: Ethics, Trial Processes**
Session chair: Robert M. Califf (Duke University)

➤ **Session Objectives:**
  ○ Spotlight and differentiate real and perceived policy barriers to the greater use of LSTs.
  ○ Highlight examples of ways in which these have been dealt with (or overcome).
  ○ Anticipate potential policy issues as trials move to leverage electronic systems.
  ○ Suggest components of a policy framework that would facilitate LSTs.

➤ **Presentations:**
  ○ **Policy overview**
    Robert M. Califf (Duke University)
  ○ **Ethical issues of bringing research and care closer together**
    Ruth R. Faden (Johns Hopkins University)
  ○ **Trial process challenges (privacy, institutional review boards)**
    Deven McGraw (Center for Democracy and Technology)

➤ **Session Questions:**
  1. What are the major policy barriers to the more widespread performance of LSTs? How have these barriers been overcome in the past? What are the priorities for change going forward?
  2. What are the important ethical issues to consider in bringing research and care closer together? What are the components of a new ethical framework to support a learning health system?
  3. What are the major privacy and human subjects research policy-associated considerations for LSTs? How have these challenges been overcome? What are the priorities for change going forward?
  4. What are the relevant ethical and policy considerations associated with randomization without additional consent in situations of equipoise?

Q&A and Open Discussion

12:00 pm   **Lunch Keynote**
             Randomized Evaluations of Accepted Choices in Treatment (REACT) trials
             Tjeerd-Pieter van Staa (Clinical Practice Research Datalink, United Kingdom)

➤ **Session Questions:**
  1. What are the REACT trials? What was the impetus for these trials? How do they compare to LSTs?
  2. What are the stakeholder engagement-related challenges you have faced in setting up/running these trials? How have the relevant stakeholder groups responded?
  3. What are the infrastructure-related challenges and opportunities you have faced? What role has the level of EHR adoption placed in facilitating or inhibiting them? What are the most crucial non-information technology infrastructure resources?
  4. How have you addressed concerns about the accuracy and validity of data in the electronic medical record?
  5. What are the policy-related challenges that you have faced? What are the differences between the UK and

U.S. systems that have facilitated or impeded these challenges?

6. What lessons learned or best practices would you pass along to LST investigators? What would you do differently?

Q&A and Open Discussion

1:00 pm **Policy Needs: Medical Product Regulatory Issues**
Session chair: Richard E. Kuntz (Planning Committee Co-Chair, Medtronic)

➢ **Presentations:**
  o **Trial complexity**
    Kenneth A. Getz (Tufts University)
  o **Simplifying clinical trials**
    Christopher B. Granger (Duke University)
  o **FDA perspective**
    Rachel E. Sherman (Center for Drug Evaluation and Research, U.S. Food and Drug Administration)

➢ **Session Questions:**
  1. In general, what is the optimal role of LSTs in the medical products regulatory approval pathway? Are there areas of medical product development in which LSTs are not useful?
  2. How can an understanding of those policy/regulatory issues that drive complexity in traditional RCTs and the strategies to counteract them be applied to the adoption and use of LSTs in medical products regulatory contexts?
  3. What are the real and perceived regulatory barriers hindering the development of an enhanced LST capacity?
  4. What are some near-term strategies for accelerating progress in the uptake of LSTs in the United States?
  5. What is the current thinking from the U.S. Food and Drug Administration in terms of how and when LSTs might be used without jeopardizing the medical products development process?

Q&A and Open Discussion

2:00 pm   **Break**

2:15 pm   **Strategies Going Forward**
Session chair: David L. DeMets (Planning Committee
Co-Chair, University of Wisconsin School of Public Health)

➤ **Session Objectives:**
   o Identify and discuss issues and key themes from the
       workshop.
   o Consider strategies and priorities for accelerating
       progress in the uptake of LSTs in the United States.

➤ **Brief Summaries and Key Stakeholder Perspectives from
the Workshop:**
   o Representatives from key stakeholders groups
       will provide an overview of key themes and issues
       identified from their perspectives.
     • Federal funders—Michael S. Lauer (National Heart,
        Lung, and Blood Institute)
     • Nongovernmental funders—Robert E. Ratner
        (American Diabetes Association)
     • U.S. Food and Drug Administration—Bram
        Zuckerman (Center for Devices and Radiological
        Health)
     • Centers for Medicare & Medicaid Services
        (CMS)—Rosemarie Hakim
     • Private payers—William H. Crown (Optum)
     • Industry—Peter Held (AstraZeneca)
     • Patients—Kate Ryan (National Women's Health
        Network)
     • Clinical researchers—Elizabeth A. Chrischilles
        (University of Iowa College of Public Health)

➤ **Panel Questions:**
   1. What are the themes of today's presentations and
       discussions that have resonated most strongly with
       you?
   2. Where do you see the most opportunity for the ap-
       plication of LSTs? What do you see to be the biggest
       barriers?

3. What will it take to seize these opportunities and overcome the barriers?
4. Based on the presentations and discussions, can you identify issues that need to be resolved by others before progress can be made? For example, as the lead of the Ethics and Processes section, can you identify critical needs in infrastructure or regulatory issues that need to be resolved before you can achieve your goals?
5. If you were granted one wish to move LSTs forward, what would that wish be?

Q&A and Open Discussion

4:15 pm   **Next Steps**
➤ **Session Description:** The workshop will conclude with a brief discussion and summary of next steps.

5:00 pm   **Adjourn**

Appendix B

Biographical Sketches of Speakers

Robert M. Califf, MD, is vice chancellor for clinical and translational research at Duke University and leads the Duke Translational Medicine Institute (DTMI), an organization focused on translating scientific discoveries into improved health outcomes. Before leading DTMI, he was founding director of the Duke Clinical Research Institute (DCRI), a premier academic research organization now part of DTMI. Under his leadership, the DCRI grew into an organization with more than 1,000 employees and an annual budget of more than $100 million; DTMI currently has a budget of more than $300 million. He attended Duke both as an undergraduate and for medical school, completing his residency at the University of California, San Francisco, before returning to Duke for a cardiology fellowship. An international leader in cardiovascular medicine, health outcomes, health care quality, and medical economics, he is among the most frequently cited authors in medicine.

Niteesh K. Choudhry, MD, PhD, is an internist and health services researcher whose work focuses on the clinical and economic consequences of using evidence-based therapies for the management of common chronic conditions. He is particularly interested in the design and evaluation of novel strategies to overcome barriers to treatment initiation and long-term medication adherence. His work employs a broad range of methods, including randomized policy evaluations, cost-effectiveness modeling, claims analyses, and surveys, and he regularly collaborates with large health insurers and employers to conduct his research. He has published more than 125 peer-reviewed articles in leading medical and policy journals and has won awards from AcademyHealth, the Society of General Internal Medicine, the International Society of Pharmacoeconomics and Outcomes Research, and the National Institute of Health Care Management for his research. Choudhry is an associate professor at Harvard Medical School and associate physician in the Division of Pharmacoepidemiology and Pharmacoeconomics and the Hospitalist Program at Brigham and Women's Hospital. He attended McGill University, received an MD, and completed his residency training in internal medicine at the University of Toronto and then served as chief medical resident for the Toronto General and Toronto Western Hospitals. He did his PhD in health policy at Harvard University, with a concentration in statistics and the evaluative sciences, and was a fellow in pharmaceutical policy research at Harvard Medical School. His work is funded by the Robert Wood Johnson Foundation, the Commonwealth Fund, the Aetna Foundation, CVS Caremark, the Agency for Healthcare Quality and Research, and others. Choudhry practices inpatient general internal/hospital medicine and has won numerous awards for teaching excellence.

Elizabeth A. Chrischilles, PhD, professor in the Department of Epidemiology, holds the Marvin A. and Rose Lee Pomerantz Chair in Public Health in the University of Iowa College of Public Health. Chrischilles is principal investigator of the Iowa Developing Evidence to Inform Decisions about Effectiveness (Iowa DEcIDE) Center and coinvestigator on a pragmatic trial in the National Institutes of Health Common Fund's Health Care Systems Research Collaboratory. She is also involved in cluster-randomized trials of team management interventions, prospective follow-up of prognostic cohorts, and linkage of claims data to prospective registries and cohorts and is leading a research team that is investigating multiple uses of an Internet-based personal health record designed with older adults.

William H. Crown, PhD, is group president of health economics and outcomes research and late-phase research for Optum. From 1982 to 1995, he was a faculty member at the Florence Heller Graduate School, Brandeis University, where he taught graduate courses in statistics and conducted research on the economics of aging and long-term-care policy. Prior to joining Optum, Crown was vice president of outcomes research and econometrics at Medstat, where he conducted numerous retrospective database analyses of the burden of illness associated with various diseases, particularly respiratory and mental health conditions. Crown's work in the area of depression was one of the first applications of econometric techniques in outcomes research to control for the effects of selection bias when retrospective data are used. He has 24 years' experience conducting health policy and income maintenance research for private- and public-sector clients. Crown is the author or coauthor of 4 books and more than 90 referenced journal articles, book chapters, and other publications.

P. J. Devereaux, MD, PhD, FRCP(C), obtained an MD from McMaster University. After medical school he completed a residency in internal medicine at the University of Calgary and a residency in cardiology at Dalhousie University. He then completed a PhD in clinical epidemiology at McMaster University. Devereaux holds a Heart and Stroke Foundation of Ontario Career Investigator Award. He is the head of cardiology and the Perioperative Cardiovascular Clinical Program at the Juravinski Hospital and Cancer Centre. He is also the scientific leader of the Perioperative Medicine and Surgical Research Group at the Population Health Research Institute. The focus of his clinical research is vascular complications around the time of surgery. He is undertaking several large international randomized controlled trials and observational studies addressing this issue. Devereaux has published more than 150 peer-reviewed papers and 40 editorials, book chapters, and commentaries.

Jeffrey M. Drazen, MD, joined the *New England Journal of Medicine* (NEJM) as editor-in-chief in July 2000. At NEJM, Drazen's responsibilities include oversight of all editorial content and policies. His editorial background includes service as an associate editor or editorial board member for the *Journal of Clinical Investigation,* the *American Journal of Respiratory Cell and Molecular Biology,* and the *American Journal of Medicine.* A specialist in pulmonology, Drazen maintains an active research program. Drazen has published more than 300 articles on topics such as lung physiology and the mechanisms involved in asthma. In 1999, he delivered the Amberson Lecture, the major research address at the annual meeting of the American Thoracic Society. In 2000, he received the Chadwick Medal from the Massachusetts Thoracic Society for his contributions to the study of lung disease. Drazen is the Distinguished Parker B. Francis Professor of Medicine at Harvard Medical School, professor of physiology at the Harvard School of Public Health, and a senior physician at Brigham and Women's Hospital. In 2003, he was elected a member of the Institute of Medicine. Drazen has served on numerous committees for the National Institutes of Health, including the Respiratory and Applied Physiology Study Section; the Lung Biology and Pathology Study Section; the Pulmonary Disease Advisory Council; the National Heart, Lung, and Blood Institute Advisory Council; the Public Access Working Group; and the National Heart, Lung, and Blood Institute's Division of Lung Disease Executive Planning Committee. He has also served on the National Research Advisory Committee of the U.S. Department of Veterans Affairs. He currently serves on the Global Initiative for Asthma Science Committee and the World Health Organization's

Scientific Advisory Group on Clinical Trials Registration and co-chairs the Institute of Medicine's Forum on Drug Discovery, Development, and Translation. Drazen earned a bachelor's degree and graduated summa cum laude from Tufts University. He received a medical degree from Harvard Medical School and completed an internship and residency at Peter Bent Brigham Hospital in Boston, Massachusetts. Drazen has received honorary degrees from the University of Ferrara in Italy, and the National and Kapodistrian University of Athens in Greece.

Ruth R. Faden, PhD, MPH, is the Philip Franklin Wagley Professor of Biomedical Ethics and director of the Johns Hopkins Berman Institute. She is also a senior research scholar at the Kennedy Institute of Ethics, Georgetown University. Faden is the author and editor of many books and articles on biomedical ethics and health policy, including *Social Justice: The Moral Foundations of Public Health and Health Policy* (with Madison Powers), *A History and Theory of Informed Consent* (with Tom L. Beauchamp), *AIDS, Women and the Next Generation* (Ruth R. Faden, Gail Geller, and Madison Powers, eds.), and *HIV, AIDS and Childbearing: Public Policy, Private Lives* (Ruth R. Faden and Nancy Kass, eds.). Faden is a member of the Institute of Medicine and a fellow of the Hastings Center and the American Psychological Association. She has served on numerous national advisory committees and commissions, including the President's Advisory Committee on Human Radiation Experiments, which she chaired. She is a co-founder of the Hinxton Group, a global community committed to advancing ethical and policy challenges in stem cell science, and the Second Wave project, an effort to ensure that the health interests of pregnant women are fairly represented in biomedical research and drug and device policies. Faden was the recipient of Lifetime Achievement Awards from the American Society for Bioethics and Humanities and from Public Responsibility in Medicine and Research in 2011. Faden's current research focuses on questions of social justice in public policy and global health. She also works on ethical challenges in biomedical science and in women's health. Faden's work in social justice is concentrated on justice theory and national and global challenges in learning health care systems, health systems design and priority setting, and access to the benefits of global investments in biomedical research.

Ryan E. Ferguson, ScD, MPH, is the acting director of the Cooperative Studies Program Coordinating Center of the U.S. Department of Veterans Affairs (VA) in Boston, Massachusetts, where he is involved in the conduct of large multicenter randomized clinical trials. He also currently serves as the program director for the VA Point of Care Research Initiative. Ferguson joined the Cooperative Studies Program in 2001 and has since focused on clinical trial methodologies for conducting pragmatic comparative effectiveness trials. In addition to the conduct of trials, his research interests include general clinical trials methodology, Bayesian statistics, renal epidemiology, molecular and genetic epidemiology, and translational research. Ferguson's published work includes first-author publications, abstracts, and presentations and a book chapter (currently in press). Ferguson is on the faculty at the Boston University School of Public Health, where he is assistant professor of epidemiology. He is also a member of the Society for Clinical Trials, the Society for Epidemiologic Research, and the American Statistical Association.

Kenneth A. Getz, MBA, is the director of sponsored research programs and research assistant professor at the Tufts Center for the Study of Drug Development, where he studies research and development management practices; pharmaceutical and biotechnology company operating models; and global investigative site, outsourcing, and study volunteer practices, trends, and policies. Getz is also the chairman of Center for Information & Study on Clinical Research Participation, a nonprofit organization that he founded to educate and raise public awareness of the clinical research enterprise, and the founder and owner of CenterWatch, a leading publisher in the clinical trials industry. A well-known speaker at conferences, symposia, universities, and corporations, Getz has published extensively in peer-reviewed journals, the trade press, and books. He holds a number of board appointments in the private and public sectors; is on the editorial boards of *Contemporary Clinical Trials*, *Research Practitioner*, the *Drug Information Journal*, and *Pharmaceutical Medicine*; and writes a column for *Applied Clinical Trials* that was a 2010 Neal Award finalist. Getz received an MBA from the J.L. Kellogg Graduate School of Management at Northwestern University and a bachelor's degree, Phi Beta Kappa, from Brandeis University. Prior to founding CenterWatch, Getz worked for more than 7 years in management consulting, where he assisted biopharmaceutical companies with the development and implementation of business strategies to improve clinical development performance.

Alan S. Go, MD, completed his internal medicine training and a general internal medicine fellowship in clinical research at the University of California, San Francisco (UCSF), before joining the Kaiser Permanente Northern California Division of Research in 1998. He is currently chief of the Cardiovascular and Metabolic Conditions Section, director of the Comprehensive Clinical Research Unit, and regional medical director of clinical trials through the Kaiser Permanente Northern California Division of Research. He is also associate professor in the Departments of Epidemiology, Biostatistics, and Medicine at UCSF and consulting professor in the Department of Health Research and Policy at the Stanford University School of Medicine. Go is also chair of the American Heart Association Epidemiology and Prevention Council's Statistics and Stroke Statistics Committee. Go is a clinical epidemiologist, outcomes researcher, and clinical trialist in the areas of cardiovascular and renal disease. He also leads several large multicenter cohort studies in these areas, including the National Heart, Lung, and Blood Institute–sponsored Cardiovascular Research Network (CVRN), a research consortium of 14 health plans in the United States. He is principal investigator of the ATRIA-CVRN Study of >34,000 adults with incident atrial fibrillation and the CVRN PRESERVE cohort of >30,000 adults with heart failure and documented systolic function. Go also leads several prospective cohort studies, including the National Institute of Diabetes and Digestive and Kidney Diseases–sponsored Assessment, Serial Assessment, and Subsequent Sequelae of Acute Kidney Injury Study and Chronic Renal Insufficiency Cohort Study. Go's current research interests include optimizing stroke prevention strategies for atrial fibrillation, the epidemiology and outcomes of heart failure with preserved versus reduced systolic function, improving the quality of care for primary and secondary prevention of cardiovascular diseases, the genetics of cardiovascular diseases, and delineating the roles of acute kidney injury and chronic kidney disease in influencing cardiovascular and renal-related adverse events.

Christopher B. Granger, MD, FACC, FAHA, is a professor of medicine in the Division of Cardiology at Duke University and director of the Cardiac Care Unit for the Duke University Medical Center. Granger is a fellow of the American College of Cardiology (ACC), the American Heart Association (AHA), and the European Society of Cardiology. He is associate editor of the *American Heart Journal* and serves on the editorial board of the *Journal of the American College of Cardiology.* He is a cardiology section author for *Current Medical Diagnosis and Treatment.* He serves on the publication oversight committee of the American Heart Association, and he is chairman of the Advisory Working Group of the American Heart Association Mission: Lifeline program. He is a member of the 2011 ACC/AHA ST-Elevation Myocardial Infarction Guidelines Committee. He has served on U.S. Food and Drug Administration advisory committees on an ad hoc basis. He is on the Board of External Experts of the National Heart, Lung, and Blood Institute. Granger's primary research interest is in the conduct and methodology of large randomized clinical trials in heart disease; he has coauthored more than 400 peer-reviewed articles. He currently serves on a number of clinical trial steering committees and data safety monitoring committees. He has coordinated the Duke Clinical Research Institute's activities in many clinical trials evaluating acute myocardial infarction (MI) reperfusion and antithrombotic strategies in acute coronary syndromes and in atrial fibrillation. Granger is co-chair of the Steering Committee of the

ARISTOTLE trial assessing an oral factor Xa inhibitor for stroke prevention in atrial fibrillation. In addition, he is co-director of the Reperfusion of Acute Myocardial Infarction in Carolina Emergency Departments projects and North Carolina statewide programs to improve reperfusion care for acute MI and care for cardiac arrest.

Rosemarie Hakim, PhD, is a senior research advisor at the Centers for Medicare & Medicaid Services (CMS). She has worked extensively with CMS staff and with the public on coverage with evidence development and CMS's clinical trial policy. She currently works with researchers to develop projects related to coverage, CED, and postcoverage analyses using CMS claims and registry data. She has developed and overseen multiple studies that have used CMS data. She has a doctorate in epidemiology from the Johns Hopkins Bloomberg School of Public Health and has extensive experience in observational study design and analysis, clinical trial design and analysis, and evidence development.

Peter Held, MD, PhD, FACC, is currently a medical science director leading an AstraZeneca effort to improve the conduct and delivery of the company's large clinical outcome studies. He is currently responsible for a number of global ongoing or planned global studies in the cardiovascular and respiratory fields. He has long experience from and interest in the methodology and conduct of both traditionally run and simplified trials. During the late 1980s he spent time at the National Heart, Lung, and Blood Institute as a visiting scientist and project officer involved in the planning and conduct of mortality/morbidity trials in heart failure and atherosclerosis. Since 1993 he has been employed by AstraZeneca Research and Development and is based in Gothenburg, Sweden. He has designed and led many global clinical development programs with a large number of new chemical entities that have led to the successful demonstration of benefit and that have resulted in regulatory approval. A scholar from the Universities of Uppsala, Linköping, and Göteborg in Sweden, he received an MD and a PhD in the mid-1980s. He specialized in cardiology and internal medicine and was appointed associate professor of cardiology in 1989. He was an adjunct professor of clinical cardiovascular research at the University of Gothenburg from 2001 to 2010.

Ralph I. Horwitz, MD, MACP, is senior vice president for clinical evaluation sciences and senior advisor to the chair of research and development at GlaxoSmithKline (GSK) and is the Harold H. Hines, Jr., Professor Emeritus of Medicine and Epidemiology at Yale University. Horwitz trained in internal medicine at institutions (the Royal Victoria Hospital of McGill University and the Massachusetts General Hospital) where science and clinical medicine were connected effortlessly. These experiences as a resident unleashed a deep interest in clinical research training, which he pursued as a fellow in the Robert Wood Johnson Clinical Scholars Program at Yale under the direction of Alvan R. Feinstein. He joined the Yale faculty in 1978 and remained there for 25 years as codirector of the Clinical Scholars Program and later as chair of the Department of Medicine. Before joining GSK, Horwitz was chair of medicine at Stanford and dean of Case Western Reserve Medical School. He is an elected member of the Institute of Medicine of the National Academy of Sciences, the American Society for Clinical Investigation, the American Epidemiological Society, and the Association of American Physicians (for which he was president in 2010). He was a member of the Advisory Committee to the National Institutes of Health director (under both Elias Zerhouni and Francis Collins). Horwitz served on the American Board of Internal Medicine and was chair in 2003. He is a master of the American College of Physicians.

Rebecca Daniels Kush, PhD, is founder, president, and chief executive officer of the Clinical Data Interchange Standards Consortium, a nonprofit standards-developing organization with a mission to develop and support global, platform-independent standards that enable information system interoperability to improve medical research and related areas of health care and a vision of "informing patient care and safety through higher quality medical research." Kush has more than 25 years of experience in the area of clinical research, including positions with the U.S. National Institutes of Health, academia, a global contract research organization, and biopharmaceutical companies in the United States and Japan. She earned a doctorate in physiology and pharmacology from the University of California, San Diego, School of Medicine. She is the lead author on the book *eClinical Trials: Planning and Implementation* and has authored numerous publications for journals, including the *New England Journal of Medicine* and *Science Translational Medicine*. She developed the Prescription Education Program for elementary and middle schools and in 2008 was named in *PharmaVoice* as one of the 100 most inspiring individuals in the life sciences industry. Kush has served on the boards of directors for the U.S. Health Information Technology Standards Panel, the Drug Information Association, and currently, Health Level 7; and she was a member of the advisory committee for the World Health Organization International Clinical Trials Registry Platform. Kush served on the appointed Planning Committee for the Office of the National Coordinator for Health Information Technology of the U.S. Department of Health and Human Services–sponsored workshop series the Digital Infrastructure for the Learning Health System for the Institute of Medicine (IOM) of National Academy of Sciences and has presented at other IOM meetings. She is a member of the National Cancer Advisory

Board Information Technology Workgroup and was invited to represent research as an appointed member of the U.S. Health Information Technology Standards Committee. Kush has developed a course, A Global Approach to Accelerating Medical Research, and has been a keynote speaker at numerous conferences in this arena in Australia, Brazil, China, Europe, Japan, South Korea, and the United States.

Carole M. Lannon, MD, MPH, is board certified in pediatrics and internal medicine and has a master's in epidemiology. She is nationally recognized for her expertise in improvement science and systems improvement. She is director of the Learning Networks Core of the James M. Anderson Center for Health Systems Excellence at the Cincinnati Children's Hospital Medical Center, professor of pediatrics at the University of Cincinnati, and senior quality advisor for the American Board of Pediatrics. Lannon is the design and implementation lead for several results-oriented, outcomes-focused improvement networks, including the Ohio Perinatal Quality Collaborative and the National Pediatric Cardiology Quality Improvement Collaborative. Lannon is principal investigator of the pediatric Center for Education and Research in Therapeutics, funded by the Agency for Healthcare Research and Quality. She is former associate editor of the *Journal of Quality and Safety in Healthcare*. She played a lead role in the design and start-up of improvement initiatives for the American Academy of Pediatrics and the National Initiative for Children's Healthcare Quality.

Michael S. Lauer, MD, is the director of the Division of Cardiovascular Sciences at the National Heart, Lung, and Blood Institute (NHLBI), part of the National Institutes of Health. In this position, Lauer provides leadership for the institute's national program for research on the causes, prevention, and treatment of cardiovascular (basic, clinical, population, and health sciences) diseases. Lauer joined NHLBI in July 2007. Lauer's primary research interests include cardiovascular clinical epidemiology and comparative effectiveness, with a focus on diagnostic testing. He also has a strong background in leadership of the cardiovascular community and longstanding interests in medical editing—for 7 years he was a contributing editor for *Journal of the American Medical Association*—and human subjects protection. Prior to joining NHLBI, Lauer served as the director of the Cleveland Clinic Foundation Exercise Laboratory and vice chair of the clinic's institutional review board. He also served as co-director of the Coronary Intensive Care Unit and director of clinical research in the clinic's Department of Cardiology. Lauer earned a bachelor of science degree in biology, summa cum laude, from the Rensselaer Polytechnic Institute in 1983 and a doctor of medicine, magna cum laude, from Albany Medical College in 1985. Following internal medical training at the Massachusetts

General Hospital, Harvard Medical School, he completed a clinical fellowship in cardiology at the Boston Beth Israel Hospital, Harvard Medical School. His further training in epidemiology included a research fellowship at NHLBI's Framingham Heart Study, Boston University; the program in clinical effectiveness, Harvard School of Public Health, Harvard University; and the Program for Physician Educators, Harvard Macy Institute. Lauer is an elected fellow of the American College of Cardiology and the American Heart Association and has been elected to membership in the American Society for Clinical Investigation. He also served as chairman of the Exercise, Cardiac Rehabilitation, and Prevention Committee of the American Heart Association's Council of Clinical Cardiology and has received numerous awards in recognition of his scientific and teaching accomplishments.

JoAnn E. Manson, MD, DrPH, is chief of the Division of Preventive Medicine at Brigham and Women's Hospital and the Michael and Lee Bell Professor of Women's Health at Harvard Medical School. She is an endocrinologist, epidemiologist, and expert in preventive medicine. She leads several major research studies addressing prevention of heart disease, diabetes, and cancer, including the VITamin D and omegA 3 triaL (VITAL; www. vitalstudy.org); the Women's Health Initiative Clinical Center in Boston, Massachusetts; the Women's Antioxidant and Folic Acid Cardiovascular Study; the cardiovascular component of the Nurses' Health Study; and the KEEPS center in Boston. Her primary research interests include the role of lifestyle and nutritional factors, particularly vitamin D, omega 3s, and folate, in the prevention of chronic disease, the effects of moderate-intensity versus vigorous exercise, and the risks and benefits of estrogen therapy. Manson has received numerous awards and honors, including the Woman in Science Award from the American Medical Women's Association, the American Heart Association's Population Research Prize, the American Heart Association's Distinguished Scientist Award, and election to the Institute of Medicine and the Association of American Physicians, and she serves as president of the North American Menopause Society. She has published more than 700 articles in the medical literature and is the author or editor of several books, including *Prevention of Myocardial Infarction* (1996), *Clinical Trials in Heart Disease* (2004), *The 30-Minute Fitness Solution* (2001), and *Hot Flashes, Hormones, & Your Health* (2007).

Deven McGraw, JD, is the director of the Health Privacy Project at the Center for Democracy and Technology (CDT). The project is focused on the development and promotion of workable privacy and security protections for electronic personal health information. McGraw is active in efforts to advance the adoption and implementation of health information technology and electronic health information exchange to improve health care.

She was one of three persons appointed by Kathleen Sebelius, the secretary of the U.S. Department of Health and Human Services (HHS), to serve on the Health Information Technology Policy Committee, a federal advisory committee established in the American Recovery and Reinvestment Act of 2009. She also served on two key workgroups of the American Health Information Community, the federal advisory body established by HHS in the George W. Bush Administration to develop recommendations on how to facilitate the use of health information technology to improve health. Specifically, she cochaired the Confidentiality, Privacy and Security Workgroup and was a member of the Personalized Health Care Workgroup. She also served on the Policy Steering Committee of the eHealth Initiative and now serves on its Leadership Committee. She is also on the Steering Group of the Markle Foundation's Connecting for Health multistakeholder initiative. McGraw has a strong background in health care policy. Prior to joining CDT, McGraw was the chief operating officer of the National Partnership for Women & Families, providing strategic direction and oversight for all of the organization's core program areas, including the promotion of initiatives to improve health care quality. McGraw was also an associate in the public policy group at Patton Boggs, LLP, and in the health care group at Ropes & Gray. She also served as deputy legal counsel to the governor of Massachusetts and taught in the Federal Legislation Clinic at the Georgetown University Law Center. McGraw graduated magna cum laude from the University of Maryland. She earned a JD, magna cum laude, and an LLM from Georgetown University Law Center and was executive editor of the *Georgetown Law Journal*. She also has a master of public health from the Johns Hopkins School of Hygiene and Public Health.

John J. Orloff, MD, is the chief medical officer and senior vice president of global development for Novartis Pharmaceuticals. In this position, Orloff is responsible for providing strategic and scientific leadership for all processes within global development and for representing Novartis externally in various forums interfacing with the scientific, academic, and health policy communities. In addition, Orloff serves as chair of the Pharma Portfolio Stewardship Board, which oversees safety and risk management plans for products within Pharma. Orloff has held a number of roles with increasing responsibility at Novartis, including section head for Bone Metabolism in Clinical Development, vice president and therapeutic area head of the Arthritis, Bone Metabolism, and Women's Health Division within Clinical Development and Medical Affairs, and most recently, head of U.S. Medical and Drug Regulatory Affairs. Orloff graduated from Dartmouth College, received a medical degree from the University of Vermont, and completed specialty training in endocrinology and metabolism at Yale University, where he served on the faculty as an associate professor of medicine before moving on to Merck Research Labs to lead clinical programs in bone metabolism.

Richard Platt, MD, MSc, is professor and chair of the Harvard Medical School Department of Population Medicine at the Harvard Pilgrim Health Care Institute. He is principal investigator of the U.S. Food and Drug Administration's (FDA's) Mini-Sentinel program and of contracts with FDA's Center for Drug Evaluation and Research and Center for Biologics Evaluation and Research to conduct postmarketing studies of the safety and effectiveness of drugs and biologics. Platt is also principal investigator of a Centers for Disease Control and Prevention (CDC) Prevention Epicenter, a CDC Center of Excellence in Public Health Informatics, and an Agency for Healthcare Research and Quality Health Maintenance Organization Research Network Developing Evidence to Inform Decisions about Effectiveness Center. He chaired the FDA Drug Safety and Risk Management Advisory Committee and is a member of the Association of American Medical Colleges' Advisory Panel on Research. Platt was co-chair of the Board of Scientific Counselors of the CDC Center for Infectious Diseases. Additionally, he chaired the National Institutes of Health study section Epidemiology and Disease Control 2 and the CDC Office of Health Care Partnerships steering committee.

Robert E. Ratner, MD, is chief scientific and medical officer for the American Diabetes Association, the nation's largest voluntary health organization leading the fight to Stop Diabetes®. Ratner joined the Association in May 2012 and provides leadership and oversight of scientific and medical activities, including research, clinical affairs, program recognition and certification, medical information, and professional education. In this capacity, he oversees the Association's support of a broad range of professional education activities and the development of the American Diabetes Association Clinical Practice Recommendations, clinical consensus reports, and expert opinions. In 2011, the Association provided $34.6 million in research funds, funding more than 400 grants at 139 leading U.S. research institutions. Prior to joining the American Diabetes Association, Ratner was a professor of medicine at Georgetown University Medical School and senior research scientist at the MedStar Health Research Institute in metropolitan Washington, DC. He recently completed a sabbatical as a Robert Wood Johnson Foundation Health Policy Fellow, having served as the study director for the Institute of Medicine Comparative Effectiveness Research Priorities Committee and a program examiner for health reform in the Health Division of the U.S. Office of Management and Budget. He received an MD from the Baylor College of Medicine in Houston, Texas, where he also completed his internal medicine training. He underwent fellowship training in endocrinology and metabolism at Harvard Medical School and the Joslin Diabetes Center in Boston, Massachusetts. He recently completed 6 years of service on the Steering Committee of the National Diabetes Education Program, representing the American Diabetes Association. He has served on the Board of Directors of the National Certification Board for Diabetes Education and the American Association of Diabetes Educators and is past president of the Washington, DC, area affiliate of the American Diabetes Association. He has served as the chair of the Government Relations Committee and the Pregnancy Council of the American Diabetes Association. He was a principal investigator for the Diabetes Prevention Program (DPP) and DPP Outcomes Study of the National Institutes of Health and served on the Steering Committee for the project nationwide. At Georgetown University, he served on the University Research Committee and cochaired the Joint Oversight Committee for Clinical Research. He was an associate editor of the *Journal of Clinical Endocrinology and Metabolism*. His research interests include diabetes therapeutics and complications, with an emphasis on translational efforts from controlled trials into community-based practice. He is the author of more than 130 original scientific articles and 20 book chapters.

Nancy Roach founded Fight Colorectal Cancer (Fight CRC) in 2005, 9 years after her mother-in-law was diagnosed with colorectal cancer. Recognizing the need for an advocacy organization, she established Fight CRC to provide focus, infrastructure, and support for colorectal cancer survivors, caregivers, and those touched by the disease. Since then, Roach has played a vital role in championing the need for a cure for colon and rectal cancer through screening, awareness, and research. Her efforts as an advocate have supported education and support for patients as well as the research community. Her leadership and passion have fostered a community of advocates supporting state and federal policies that have led to increased colorectal cancer research opportunities across the country. Over the last 4 years, Fight CRC has directed more than $250,000 in research funding to young investigators. Roach currently serves as the chair of the Board of Directors and serves on the National Cancer Institute (NCI) Board of Scientific Counselors and the Clinical Trial and Translational Research Advisory Committee. She is on the Executive Committee of the Clinical Trials Transformation Initiative, a U.S. Food and Drug Administration–Duke University public–private partnership, and is a past chair of its Finance Committee. She has been involved with cooperative groups and SPORES and currently serves on the NCI Colon Task Force. She served on the U.S. Department of Defense congressionally directed Medical Research Program Integration Panel in 2010, the first year that colorectal cancer research was funded by the program. She is a past chair of the NCI Patient Advocate

Steering Committee and received the NCI Director's Service Award when she stepped down. She has also received the Preventing Colorectal Cancer Champion Award and the Colon Cancer Alliance Sapphire Visionary Award, in recognition of her efforts on behalf of patients. She has spoken on behalf of patients at meetings such as the American Association for Cancer Research, the Friends of Cancer Research/Brookings Institution Conference on Clinical Research, and the Oxford University-Duke University-McMaster University Sensible Guidelines for Clinical Trials.

Kate Ryan, MPA, is the senior program coordinator at the National Women's Health Network (NWHN). In this role, she is responsible for developing and implementing a program of legislative and regulatory advocacy that focuses on reducing women's exposure to unnecessary drug and medical treatment risks. Ryan leads advocacy efforts to increase research on women's health and increase women's participation in clinical trials and health research. Through work with the National Institute of Child Health and Human Development and the U.S. Food and Drug Administration, Ryan brings women's voices to the health policy debates in Washington, DC, and the states and advocates for a health care system that is accessible to all and meets the needs of diverse women. Prior to joining the NWHN, Ryan worked in the Capitol Hill office of U.S. Representative Joe Sestak (D-PA), where she worked on health care reform and the women's issues portfolio and managed a variety of constituent services programs. Before moving to Washington, DC, Ryan volunteered in Ghana with the Alliance for Reproductive Health Rights to monitor and assess the availability of and access to women's sexual and reproductive health services under the Ghanaian National Health Insurance Scheme. As part of this work, Ryan also monitored Ghana's progress on Millennium Development Goals 4 and 5: to reduce child mortality and improve maternal health. Ryan received an MPA in international public and nonprofit management and policy analysis with a focus on women's rights from the New York University Wagner Graduate School of Public Service.

Lewis G. Sandy, MD, is senior vice president for clinical advancement of UnitedHealth Group (a Fortune 25 diversified health and well-being company dedicated to helping people live healthier lives). At UnitedHealth Group, he focuses on clinical innovation, payment/delivery reforms to modernize the U.S. health care system, and physician collaboration. He also is a principal in the UnitedHealth Center for Health Reform and Modernization, with a focus on payment/delivery innovation and policy. From 2003 to 2007, he was executive vice president and chief medical officer of UnitedHealthcare, UnitedHealth Group's largest business, focusing on the employer/individual health benefits market. From 1997 to 2003, he was executive vice president of the Robert Wood Johnson Foundation (RWJF). At RWJF, he was responsible for the Foundation's program development and management, strategic planning, and administrative operations. Prior to this, Sandy was a program vice president of the Foundation, focusing on the Foundation's workforce, health policy, and chronic care initiatives. An internist and former health center medical director at the Harvard Community Health Plan in Boston, Massachusetts, Sandy received BS and MD degrees from the University of Michigan and an MBA degree from Stanford University. A former RWJF Clinical Scholar and Clinical Fellow in Medicine at the University of California, San Francisco, Sandy served his internship and residency at the Beth Israel Hospital in Boston. He is a senior fellow of the Department of Health Policy and Management, University of Minnesota School of Public Health.

Joe V. Selby, MD, MPH, is the first executive director of the Patient-Centered Outcomes Research Institute (PCORI). A family physician, clinical epidemiologist, and health services researcher, he has more than 35 years of experience in patient care, research, and administration. He identifies strategic issues and opportunities for PCORI and implements and administers programs authorized by the PCORI Board of Governors. Building on the work of the Board and interim staff, Selby leads the organizational development of PCORI, which was established by Congress through the 2010 Patient Protection and Affordable Care Act. In addition to creating an organizational structure to carry out a national research agenda, Selby leads PCORI's external communications, including work to establish effective two-way communication channels with the public and stakeholders about PCORI's work. Selby joined PCORI from Kaiser Permanente, Northern California, where he was director of the Division of Research for 13 years and oversaw a department of more than 50 investigators and 500 research staff working on more than 250 ongoing studies. He was with Kaiser Permanente for 27 years. An accomplished researcher, Selby has authored more than 200 peer-reviewed articles and continues to conduct research, primarily in the areas of diabetes outcomes and quality improvement. His publications cover a spectrum of topics, including effectiveness studies of colorectal cancer screening strategies; treatment effectiveness, population management, and disparities in diabetes mellitus; primary care delivery; and quality measurement. Selby was elected to membership in the Institute of Medicine in 2009 and was a member of the Agency for Healthcare Research and Quality Study Section for Health Care Quality and Effectiveness from 1999 to 2003. A native of Fulton, Missouri, Selby received a medical degree from Northwestern University and a master's in public health from the University of California, Berkeley. He was a commissioned officer in the Public Health Service from 1976 to 1983 and received the Commissioned Officer's Award in 1981. He serves as a lecturer in the Department of Epidemiology and Biostatistics, University of California, San Francisco, School of Medicine, and as a consulting professor in health research and policy at the Stanford University School of Medicine. Selby was appointed PCORI executive director on May 16, 2011, and formally began his duties on July 1, 2011.

Rachel E. Sherman, MD, MPH, is the associate director for medical policy, Center for Drug Evaluation and Research (CDER), U.S. Food and Drug Administration (FDA). She is responsible for developing, implementing, and coordinating medical policy programs and strategic initiatives, including regulation of prescription drug promotion and advertising, through the Center's Division of Drug Marketing, Advertising, and Communications. Sherman provides leadership and scientific guidance and advice in clinical trial implementation and facilitates the development and implementation of agency policy related to human subject protection and good clinical practices through the development of regulations, guidance documents, and procedures related to medical policy issues. Key activities involve leveraging of resources and expertise from within FDA and from industry, academia, and other federal agencies to achieve agency goals. Sherman is leading the agency's implementation of the Sentinel Initiative and the development and implementation of biosimilars policy. Sherman began her career with FDA in the Division of Antiviral Drug Products in CDER in 1989. During her tenure there, both as a medical reviewer and as a team leader, she played a pivotal role in the rapid development of new agents to treat human immunodeficiency virus infection and other viral diseases. Since 1998, she has held a series of senior management positions in the agency, including deputy office director for the Office of Drug Evaluation I, deputy office director of the Office of Medical Policy in CDER, and associate commissioner for clinical programs. From 2003 until her return to CDER in 2009, Sherman directed the Office of Critical Path Programs in the Office of the Commissioner, leading FDA's Critical Path Initiative, an agency initiative to spur innovation and foster efforts to modernize the way in which FDA-regulated products are developed, evaluated, manufactured, and used. Sherman is a board-certified internist and infectious disease subspecialist. She received an AB in mathematics from Washington University, an MD from the Mt. Sinai School of Medicine, and an MPH from the Johns Hopkins School of Hygiene and Public Health.

Elsie M. Taveras, MD, MPH, is an associate professor of population medicine at Harvard Medical School and associate professor of pediatrics at Children's Hospital Boston. She received bachelor of science and medical doctor degrees from New York University in New York City. After receiving an MD, she did her internship, residency, and chief residency at the Boston Combined Residency Program in Pediatrics, a joint program of Children's Hospital Boston and Boston Medical Center. In 2001, Taveras joined the Harvard Pediatric Health Services Research Fellowship Program and received a master's in public health with a concentration in clinical effectiveness from the Harvard School of Public Health. Taveras is the co-director of the Obesity Prevention Program at the Department of Population Medicine. Taveras is also on staff at Children's Hospital Boston, where she directs a multidisciplinary childhood obesity prevention clinic in general pediatrics. Taveras's main focus of research is understanding determinants of obesity in children and adolescents and developing interventions across the life course to prevent obesity in children, especially in underserved populations. Taveras's publications have examined diet, activity, sleep, and weight determinants in later childhood and origins of obesity early in life in young children.

Tjeerd-Pieter van Staa, MD, PhD, MSc, MA, studied medicine and received a medical degree in 1987 at the Erasmus University of Rotterdam, Rotterdam, the Netherlands. After several years of working as a practicing physician, he joined the pharmaceutical industry and worked as an epidemiologist and was also the European qualified person for drug safety. During this time, he obtained an MSc in epidemiology (McGill University, Canada) and was awarded a PhD in pharmacoepidemiology at Utrecht University, Utrecht, the Netherlands, in 1999. He also has an MA in medical law and ethics. In 2006, he joined the Medicines and Healthcare Products Regulatory Agency as director of research of the Clinical Practice Research Datalink (CPRD; the General Practice Research Database [GPRD] is part of CPRD). He has published more than 130 peer-reviewed articles and is a well-recognized speaker in the field of pharmacoepidemiology, pharmacovigilance, and osteoporosis. He has been awarded several academic affiliations (Utrecht University; Medical Research Council, Southampton, United Kingdom) and is honorary professor at the London School of Hygiene and Tropical Medicine. van Staa is the recipient of the 2005 Iain I Boyle Award of the European Calcified Tissue Society (which consists of a monetary award to the scientist who has made significant contributions to bone disease research [http://www.ectsoc.org]). His current research activities concern the implementation of randomized clinical trials that use routinely collected electronic health records (as outlined in a recent article in the *British Medical Journal*). Two cluster trials (on randomization practices) and a large pharmacogenetic study within GPRD are close to completion. van Staa is also involved in the implementation of multiple linkages of GPRD to other health care data sets, including cancer and registries, cardiovascular disease registries, air pollution, and bowel screening data. Visualization and evaluation of data quality are other research interests.

James B. Young, MD, is professor of medicine and executive dean of the Cleveland Clinic Lerner College of Medicine of Case Western Reserve University and chair of the Endocrinology and Metabolism Institute. He is also physician director of institutional relations and development and a medical director of the Kaufman Center for Heart Failure. He holds the George and Linda Kaufman Chair and is the study chairman of the National Institutes of Health, U.S. Food and Drug Administration, and Centers for Medicare & Medicaid Services Interagency Registry for Mechanical Circulatory Assist Support. He has a joint appointment to the Clinic's Multiorgan Transplant Center. Young is certified as a diplomat of the American Board of Internal Medicine as well as the subspecialty of cardiovascular disease and holds medical licensure from the states of California, Illinois, Ohio, Pennsylvania, and Texas. Young spent his early years in the San Francisco, California, Bay Area and then attended the University of Kansas, where he received a bachelor of arts degree with honors in biology and was a resident of Stephenson Scholarship Hall. He matriculated to the Baylor College of Medicine in Houston, Texas, where he was awarded a medical doctor degree with honors in 1974 and was elected to the Alpha Omega Alpha medical honor society. Young remained in Houston at the Baylor Affiliated Hospitals to complete his clinical training, joining the faculty and becoming a professor of medicine with tenure in 1992. He was the clinical coordinator and scientific director for Michael E. DeBakey's Multiorgan Transplant Center at The Methodist Hospital and the Baylor College of Medicine. He subsequently relocated to the Cleveland Clinic in Ohio in 1995, when he became head of the Section of Heart Failure and Cardiac Transplant Medicine in the Department of Cardiovascular Disease. In 1998 Young, along with his surgical colleague, Patrick McCarthy, created the Kaufman Center for Heart Failure at the Cleveland Clinic. Young's research activities began during his residency and fellowship training when he was a Lipid Research Clinic physician. He subsequently focused his efforts on heart failure, mechanical circulatory support, and cardiac transplant therapeutics, including early experiences with dopamine receptor agonists, angiotensin-converting-enzyme inhibitors, beta blockers, calcium channel blockers, angiotensin receptor blockers, many new immunosuppressants, and a variety of parenteral inotropes and vasodilators. He has collaborated extensively with his basic science research associates, focusing on translational research with respect to the molecular biology of cardiac remodeling, allograft arteriopathy, and transplanted heart rejection. Young served as the United States principal or co–principal investigator for the HOPE, RESOLVED, SPICE, VMAC, MIRACLE-ICD, RED-HF, ACCLAIM, ONTARGET, TRANSCEND, and

CHARM multicenter clinical trials. He has participated in more than 150 clinical trials as an investigator. Young has published almost 600 articles and several textbooks. Professionally, Young is most proud of his contributions to the development and administration of donor organ procurement programs, his efforts to secure recognition for the newly emerging cardiology subspecialty of heart failure and cardiac transplant medicine, his collaborations with basic and clinical scientists, his contributions to a unique medical school curriculum, and the programs that he helped develop in Houston and Cleveland.

Bram Zuckerman, MD, is a graduate of the Boston University Medical School. He completed postgraduate training in internal medicine at Baltimore City Hospital and cardiology at the Johns Hopkins program. Prior to joining the U.S. Food and Drug Administration (FDA) in 1992, he was involved in basic research in hemodynamics at the University of Colorado Medical School and practiced noninvasive and invasive cardiology in Denver, Colorado, and Northern Virginia. He joined the FDA Division of Cardiovascular Devices (DCD) as a medical officer in 1992 and has been actively involved in the development and review of clinical trials for many new cardiovascular devices. In May 2001 he was appointed a deputy director in DCD. He was appointed to his current position as director of the FDA Division of Cardiovascular Devices in September 2002.